TABLE OF CONTENTS

preface

I feel blessed that I made the connection between food and health—two essential elements of healthy, optimal living—before ailments or disease had a chance to rob me of a good quality of life. Because I'm passionate about food and health, it tends to be the subject of many of my conversations, both personally and professionally. I have many family members who suffer from poor eating habits and chronic disease. I have nutrition students, wellness coaching clients, and wellness workshop attendees fighting the same uphill battle. I notice strangers struggling to climb stairs, to bend and lift light packages, or walk short distances when they shouldn't be. I believe the key to taking charge of your life and creating a future built on a strong body and boundless potential is making the connection between your food and your health. I know from personal experience that once you really "get" the role of food in the body and make a commitment to live your best life, the rest of the journey is simple. The struggle over what to eat ceases. The helplessness over maintaining a healthy weight vanishes. The uncertainty of how to ensure your kids have the best chance at a happy, healthy, and productive life is diminished.

Instead, what you'll feel is *empowerment.*

Quick Wins is written for busy people who care about their health and the health of their families. In this book, you'll find what I know to be the easiest and most effective strategies for making the connection between food and health. Without this connection, poor health may be unavoidable. To put it simply, if we want any shot at reclaiming a healthy future—a future all of our children deserve—we have to learn how to eat a traditional diet while living in a modern world. I'm concerned with how destructive the simple act of eating and feeding our families has become over recent decades. It's time for us to slow down, just a little bit, and refocus on nurturing our families. Until we direct some of our energy toward health, we'll simply continue to pass on our destructive eating patterns to our children.

Quick Wins provides a fresh perspective, relevant information, tools, and resources that are effective in changing the eating habits of modern families. In Chapter 10, you'll find 9 easy changes you and your family can make right now. Along the way, I've included inspirational quotes to keep you motivated, as well as "Quick Wins Tip" boxes to support your transition to healthy eating habits. You'll also find "Believe It or Not" boxes with food facts and statistics that are sure to amaze you. As you complete each chapter, you'll find a nice recap in the "Food for Thought" section. Finally, the appendices are chock-full of valuable resources, worksheets and checklists. You'll find my top picks for great cookbooks, websites and food blogs; tips and checklists for stocking a healthy pantry, easy ways to shop and eat local; a food log and journal to record your accomplishments and track your eating, and much more!

At the heart of a quality of life is not money, fame or fortune—but good health. Each of us has the power to make choices that will either add to our health or take away from it. *Quick Wins* is my way of helping you and your family make the right choices.

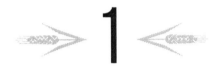

WHAT ARE QUICK WINS?

I won't lie to you: Eating healthy in America today is tough for families. As fast-paced lifestyles, two working parents, and easy access to fast food and convenience food have become the norm, healthy eating has increasingly become a global challenge for families.

There's something else I won't lie to you about: Healthier eating *is* possible for families.

> "Take the first step in faith. You don't have to see the whole staircase, just take the first step."
> **DR. MARTIN LUTHER KING JR.**

This book is designed to help you break away from societal eating trends, poor family habits, and self-limiting beliefs that contribute to chronic disease, low energy, adult and childhood obesity, and disconnected families. If you've tried to eat healthier yourself or attempted to implement better eating habits within your family, you may have gotten tired of swimming against the current and given up. Changing a lifestyle is hard! But with the right approach and the right tools, your family *can* do it—and reap the benefits of a healthier and happier life.

LOOKING FORWARD

Have you ever considered what a new, healthier life would look like? What would you or your spouse be able to accomplish that you can't do now? Do you think you would feel any different? What ailments do you have that would potentially go away? How would your children's lives benefit from a healthier start?

I've thought about these questions myself. Here's how I envision a life of good health for my family:

- My son, husband and I have strong and flexible bodies that allow us to live independently well into our senior years (i.e., without a caretaker or nurse).
- We each have a sound mind.
- We are free of disease.
- We have abundant energy.
- My husband and I are able to pass on a legacy of health to our young son and future generations.

A WINNING PHILOSOPHY

The key to developing "strong swimming skills" and improving your odds for success is what I call "Quick Wins." The principle of Quick Wins is based on implementation of a core group of health-promoting habits that yield positive results if performed systematically. Contrary to popular thinking on healthy eating, Quick Wins are designed to help you and your family be winners, not just participants, in the race for a healthy lifestyle. The difference between a participant and a winner is results. A participant is in the race but has not yet crossed the finish line. A winner is a participant who crosses the finish line and reaches success. Quick Wins are targeted toward *results*.

Success isn't attained by taking huge leaps every now and then. On the contrary, success is the sum of small steps repeated day in and day out. To successfully change your eating habits, you'll have to break free of the idea of taking giant steps. Giant steps, like becoming an overnight vegetarian, create a drastic change in your lifestyle. Without taking time to research healthy vegetarian recipes or meat alternatives, you'll be unprepared—and ultimately, unsuccessful. If the change doesn't feel comfortable and natural, odds are great that you'll quit your newfound vegetarian lifestyle before you even approach your family about switching to meatless meals.

The goal is for your family to be winners, so you can't quit halfway through the race if you want to realize your goal. You must keep going.

in a nutshell

Quick Wins are simple habits you and your family can do right now to move you toward the finish line. Quick Wins are:

1. Easy to achieve
2. Adaptable
3. Expandable
4. Momentum builders

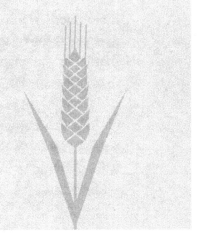

THE DIFFERENCE

How can you tell if Quick Wins are working for your family? You know Quick Wins are working when the struggle to eat better begins to subside. Actions become automatic, and results become consistent. You can sense a pull toward more nutritious eating rather than a push away from it. You hear less complaining from your kids, and more of the food you prepare is eaten.

Friends and family begin to notice something different about your skin tone, energy level or even weight. They start to associate these positive changes with the natural foods you've been bringing with you to work, the healthy menu selections you make when dining out, and the water you always seem to be drinking and carrying around with you. Your kids' behavior and grades start to improve.

The Quick Wins I share with you in this book have helped me, my family, wellness coaching clients and countless others through my seminars, workshops and radio broadcasts attain a healthier and happier life—and they can help you, too. Integrating these strategies into your everyday routine will raise your awareness, increase your knowledge, broaden your experience, and enhance your motivation to clean up your family's diet. Don't worry about trying to digest too much information all at once. At the end of each chapter in the "Food for Thought" section, you'll find a summary of the chapter's main points. Use these small nuggets of information to inspire, encourage, and jump-start your healthy eating strategies.

As you and your family cross the finish line, the pride and exhilaration will be unequaled. You'll become a family that stared overweight, obesity, and chronic disease in the face and accepted the challenge to not become victims of unhealthy living. As you experience the great feeling of victory for yourself, you'll be inspired to guide other families toward the finish line and a legacy of good health.

Simple changes, like the ones you'll start right now, equal Quick Wins for your health and the well-being of your family. An exciting journey lies before you. A future of abundant energy, excitement, and optimal health is waiting for you. Just take the first step and know the next step is right in front of you.

2

FOUR DRESS SIZES AGO

I was a chubby little kid. Full, cocoa-brown cheeks; fat, little fingers; large thighs for my size; short, stubby ponytails; and a big smile. I'm envisioning an old photo of me at age 3 in a blue-leather vest that hung over the bar in my grandmother's

kitchen for over a decade. My mom had taken great care to comb my hair into two ponytails, tied with neatly ironed white ribbons. After making sure every hair was in place and my clothes were carefully assembled, she sat me in a kitchen chair and snapped a memorable photo of a happy and loved little girl. One way our family expressed love was through food. As you can see in the photo, I was definitely a happy and loved little girl!

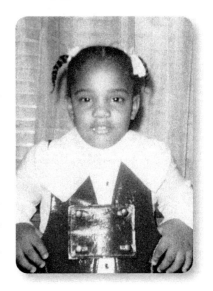

As I got older, I lost some of that "baby fat," as family members called it, but I was never what you would consider a "small" girl. I was slightly heavier than average when compared to my peers throughout middle and high school.

When I was growing up, poor body image wasn't as pervasive as it is now. My friends and I liked nice clothes and somewhat tried to keep up with current trends, but we didn't feel pressured to look thin or to wear a certain size. As teens growing up in rural North Carolina in the '80s, clothing trends included Members Only jackets, Levi jeans and T-shirts with either our names or our boyfriends' names spelled out on the back with iron-on lettering. Body size wasn't a real factor in that style of clothing. We were conscious of keeping our hair looking nice, our nails polished, and our lips shining with gloss. The rest we didn't fuss over. Today, the trend in girls' clothing is form-fitting tops and pants, making body shape and appearance more pronounced.

flawed image

The reality of growing up female in today's image-conscious society is startling. Girls today have a lot to contend with in terms of body image and self-esteem issues. In 2005, Dove beauty company reported findings from a telephone survey of 3,200 girls, aged 18 to 64, from 10 countries around globe, including Argentina, Brazil, Canada, France, Italy, Japan, Netherlands, Portugal, the UK, and the United States. The survey found that more than 90 percent of the girls included in the survey would like to change at least one aspect of their appearance, with body weight topping the list of things they would change (Campaign for Real Beauty, 2004). Twenty-five percent of those polled indicated they would consider plastic surgery to correct their perceived flaws.

In high school, I joined the junior varsity cheerleading squad. I was so excited to make the cut. A couple of close friends were on the squad, and they painted a colorful picture of camaraderie and unmeasured fun while traveling with the basketball and football teams to away games. Students who got to leave school early on game days had an air of superiority over the kids left behind; they peered out of fifth-period English and math as we jovially walked by the classrooms, headed for the buses.

Junior varsity cheerleading started out as a lot of fun, but during football season, I gradually began to feel uncomfortable in my cheerleading uniform. The skirt felt a little tight in the waistline, and I was constantly tugging at the bottom of it to pull it down. My cheerleading top wasn't fitting right either. Each time I jumped or lifted my arms to clap above my head, my top would raise high above my waist just like the other girls' tops did. The difference was that my top didn't come down naturally—it got stuck over my large breasts—so, eventually, I was constantly pulling that down, too. I felt that everyone in the stands had their eyes on me instead of the playing teams as I continuously tugged and pulled at either my skirt or top throughout each game. I became so self-conscious that I eventually quit the squad and joined the color guard in our marching band, where long black pants and loose white tops with vests were the official uniform attire.

GOODBYE HOME COOKING, HELLO FAST FOOD

Although my weight was becoming a little uncomfortable in high school, the pounds didn't really start to tip the scales toward unhealthy until the middle of my college years. For the first time, I was living by my own food rules. I didn't have access to Mom's home-cooked meals, and I had open access to all sorts of fast food and processed food from the college cafeteria and restaurants near my college campus.

Gaining weight during college, where poor eating habits are the norm, isn't uncommon. However, the impact of gaining weight after the age of 18 can have significant consequences. A 2005 study of 62,000 women, published in the journal *Cancer Epidemiology, Biomarkers & Prevention*, showed that breast cancer risk rises by 40 percent post-menopause in adult women who gain 21 to 30 pounds after the age of 18.

Twenty-one to 30 pounds may sound like a lot of weight, but it's quite easy to gain these unwanted pounds by eating a Standard American Diet. Convenient and unlimited access to fried chicken, pizza, burgers, hot dogs, macaroni and cheese, pancakes, cookies, ice cream, and other unhealthy fare easily contributes to weight gain. Don't think kids get by any better if they live off campus. Off-campus living has its own set of nutritional challenges. Students living outside of campus dormitories often have little experience in cooking and lack a basic understanding of what constitutes a healthy meal. This is one reason it's so critical for us to teach our kids, while they're young, how to make healthy food choices and how to cook basic meals.

As kids get older, teach them to grow basic herbs and vegetables and show them how to shop for nutritious foods so a knowledge of how to eat well becomes a basic life skill for them, just like learning to wash clothes and to drive. Try planting a simple container garden on your porch, on your deck, or on a table in a sunny part of your house so your kids will understand food's growth process.

When your kids are at least 6 or 7 years old, start taking them grocery shopping with

BELIEVE IT OR NOT
Freshman weight gain is a real phenomenon. Breakfast, all-you-can-eat lunch options, and excess junk food contribute unneeded pounds.

you and teach them to read food labels. However, I wouldn't advise taking kids younger than 6 on a grocery store tour unless you want your well-intended educational excursion to turn into a fit of frustration and temper tantrums. Instead, visit a local farmer's market or fruit stand to teach younger kids how to recognize a variety of whole fruits and vegetables. Learning these skills as children will benefit them greatly as adults.

"It's never too late–in fiction
or in life–to revise."
NANCY THAYER

GRADUATE SCHOOL OVERLOAD

In many ways, going straight to graduate school was a good thing. My college advisor convinced me it would be easier to complete a post-secondary degree if I continued on while I was still in the mindset of rigorous daily studying. She also assured me that working on a graduate degree without the responsibility of working a full-time job would be a luxury coveted by many of my peers. I soon learned she was right when I added a full-time teaching job to my plate while writing my thesis.

The stress of graduate school made me eat horribly. I didn't have the time or money to hang out with friends, shop or travel, so I felt the least I could do was eat whatever the heck I wanted to—when I wanted to. After a long week, my best friend and I had a weekend ritual of picking up a large Lil' Dino's pepperoni pizza and two 24-ounce Budweisers before heading to my apartment to "pig out" while we watched a good movie. I think we did this on weekends for about a year. This was a lot of food for two people of our stature. I'm 5 foot 5 inches and my best friend is 5 foot 1 inch, both with medium-sized frames. Eating a large pizza between the two of us, plus roughly 300 calories from beer, was way more food than either of our sedentary bodies needed.

A lot of times we felt eater's remorse seeping in, just like most people experience after eating way too much. The bloated, sleepy, gassy feeling reminds you that you've messed up. When you eat whatever the heck you want every now and then, it's called a splurge. When you do it every week or every day, it's considered abuse. And trust me, when you abuse your body with too much food or the wrong food, it doesn't feel good.

Where's the "Off" Button?

But self-limiting beliefs—those that keep you from doing something you want or need to do—will keep you eating when you know you should stop. These beliefs are yours alone, although they may have been created as a result of interactions with another person who had great influence in your life, like a parent or teacher.

Believing that one unhealthy indulgence wrecks the whole the day, nutritionally speaking, is an example of a common self-limiting belief. You know the story: You get invited out to lunch with friends or family when you've committed yourself to eating better. Most everyone knows that sticking to a healthy-eating regimen at a restaurant can be quite challenging, so you end up eating a few too many hot wings and potato skins on the appetizer sampler, and you down your whole plate of chicken and pasta, which you know is enough to feed two or three people. Before the check is paid, you're feeling defeated. You believe this one slip-up

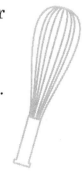

BELIEVE IT OR NOT
According to a recent Centers for Disease Control report, approximately 2.4 million more adults were obese in 2009 than in 2007. In each of the 50 states, more than 15 percent of adults are obese, and in nine states, over 30 percent of adults are obese.

gives you reason to abandon your eating goals for the rest of the day. So you turn one splurge into a full-day feeding frenzy, having a soda and chips around 3 p.m. and fried chicken for dinner. Then you *really* feel guilty and end up completely abandoning your goals of eating healthier. When you think this way, you've essentially bought into a belief system where eating a bag of chips or a bowl of ice cream, for example, is so horrible that it justifies your continuing to abuse your body by making poor eating choices that can, over time, adversely affect your health.

This is exactly the mindset I had with my Lil' Dino's pizza. As if all we had eaten weren't enough, many times I would add dessert to our menu, such as ice cream or cookies, or both. In my mind, we were treating ourselves, but in actuality, we were harming ourselves. Looking back, I can see how distorted my thinking was.

Think about it: Have you ever skipped your evening walk or workout because you figured you'd already blown it for the day with that hunk of cake you ate earlier? That form of thinking is counter-productive to good health. What if you applied that all-or-nothing mindset to other areas of your life? Say you're driving your car to work and you happen to run off the road a little bit. Do you continue to drive on the gravel and grass into the woods? No! You automatically pull your car back onto the road and keep on driving toward your destination.

Why don't we take that instinctive approach when our eating habits go off-road? If you take control of your thoughts just like you take control of your car's steering wheel, you'll begin to see the important connection between your behaviors and your health. Once you make that connection, you won't let anything stand in the way of doing what you need to do to protect your body and your health. As you'll see in the section "A New Attitude," the ability to recognize and dismiss negative thinking patterns as soon as they popped into my head helped me change my unhealthy attitude toward food and create a more positive mindset that's continually focused on health and longevity. So what if I eat too much chocolate cheesecake at lunch one day? I don't continue to abuse myself by eating more sugary food later in the day. I get over it and move on!

Quickly realigning with my health goals helps me feel good about myself and empowers me with a balanced perspective about how to enjoy food. Now that I'm a parent, a healthy approach to eating helps me instill healthy values in my son. When I feel good about myself, it shows. I'm more relaxed, cheerful, and kinder to others. I tend to have more energy and interest in doing the things I need to do to take care of myself, like making sure I get in at least eight glasses of water during the day, as well as a brisk walk. My son watches everything I do. I know that by sticking with my healthy habits, I'm being a good role model for him.

A WEIGHTY ISSUE

I believe natural, nourishing food is the foundation of good health, but as you now know, I didn't always live by this philosophy. I spent the majority of my young-adult years with thighs that rubbed together like sandpaper and a pantry with enough Snickers, Doritos, and other junk food to stock a small convenience store. My closets were overstocked, too, but with carefully chosen clothes, including loose-fitting blouses in an array of colors to camouflage my 38DD breasts.

According to one of the many online ideal body weight calculators, a healthy weight range for a medium-frame person like me standing at 5 feet 5 inches is between 111 and 150 pounds. I was at my highest weight in my 20s. In graduate school, I weighed roughly 170 pounds, about 20 pounds overweight. But as they say, hindsight is 20/20. When I look back at my life during those years, I realize I was carrying around far more than just fat. I was carrying a legacy of obesity and chronic illness.

QUICK WINS TIPS

Hectic school schedules, jobs, socializing, and lack of sleep all contribute to unhealthy eating habits among students. It's easy to make good grades *and* eat a good diet. Try these tips for starters:

1. Eat breakfast each day.

2. Drink plenty of water.

3. Never go longer than four or five hours without eating.

4. Avoid foods high in fat, sugar and salt. (See Chapter 8 for tips on limiting these culprits in your diet.)

5. Limit alcohol intake.

6. Don't eat calorie-dense foods late at night.

Most of my family, on both my mom's and dad's sides, has had an ongoing struggle with weight. So the fact that I was gradually packing on the pounds as I got older felt like a natural course of events for me. Although I felt destined to be a little on the heavy side, a part of me still felt trapped by the thought of surrendering to the same weight issues that took their toll on my mom, grandmothers, aunties, and cousins. And it wasn't just the women in my family who weighed more than they should. The men in my family also carried around extra pounds, mainly around the midsection—the least healthy place to store body fat, according to health experts.

Nevertheless, feeling stuck in a cycle of obesity and chronic illness wasn't enough to motivate me to take control and stop eating irresponsibly. In fact, for nearly two years, I had a weekly ritual of baking a pan of double-chocolate brownies to snack on each day when I got home from class or work in the microbiology lab. I remember the anticipation I felt while driving home in the evenings, of eating brownies warmed in the microwave with a glass of ice-cold milk. Once I walked through my apartment door, I couldn't drop my purse and backpack fast enough!

You would think that after eating a whole pan of brownies, I would be guilted into trying to burn off some of the excess calories, but I wasn't. Apart from taking an occasional Jazzercise class with a couple of girlfriends, I didn't exercise much. Although I did get some physical activity from going to Jazzercise, it really was more of a social outing than anything else. I rarely broke a sweat during class, and afterward my friends and I almost always rewarded ourselves with Dairy Queen ice cream. My favorite was a vanilla cone dipped in chocolate or an Oreo Blizzard. Afterward, my old self-limiting belief spoke up in a raised voice. "I deserve it," I would hear each time after the last lick of ice cream.

A NEW ATTITUDE

On a warm, sunny afternoon almost 17 years ago, I opened my front door to greet my blind date for the evening, which had been arranged by my best friend. This handsome, ex-Air Force staff sergeant standing in front of me with a gentle smile turned out to be the catalyst I needed to make some powerful changes in my life. Our relationship eventually exposed me to a new way of living that offered me a chance to be healthier and happier.

I remember how much I enjoyed our conversations. We talked for hours at a time, sitting on my living-room sofa, close to one another. We talked about history, politics, health, and everyday life experiences. Michael had traveled the world during his 10 years in the military and had a unique way of coloring his perspectives with parallels from other cultures and past events. He brought home the notion that our experiences and our choices shape the way we think and engage the world. Michael spoke passionately about his "constitution"—the guiding philosophy for living his life—which intrigued me. This concept of consciously focusing on a personal philosophy was new to me. I could look at the way he lived his life and ascertain that, among other things, personal responsibility was firmly rooted in his constitution. Seeing how Michael embraced his personal philosophies made me look more closely at my own life. I reflected upon the personal choices I had made thus far and the experiences those choices had provided me. Professionally, my life was in a good place, but other areas required more attention. It became clear that for the better part of my adult life, I had approached personal matters like my health and well-being reactively. I was adamant about getting physicals annually and seeing a doctor when I was sick, but I spent very little time thinking about my wellness philosophy. I ate the same way my friends and family did, engaged in little physical activity, and didn't give much thought to the role diet and exercise played in my health. It's funny: When the people around you are overweight and unhealthy, you don't take notice of yourself because you blend in with the crowd.

Fortunately, my health has always been good, despite the fact that I paid little attention to eating proper food or being physically active during my young adult years. My blood pressure was, and still is, within normal ranges, and I've never experienced glucose or cholesterol problems.

Michael was indeed the catalyst for my new attitude. If you recall from high school chemistry class, a catalyst is an agent that provides an alternative route of reaction under favorable conditions. Although the catalyst participates in the reaction, it is neither consumed nor changed. That's why I think of Michael as my catalyst. He was a change agent that came into my life at just the right time to facilitate a much-needed transformation. Let me be clear: He didn't ask me to change. He simply exposed me to new lifestyle choices and supported me once I decided I wanted to become a healthier and more vibrant woman.

A Closer Look

I've since created a food philosophy that serves as the guiding principle for the way I eat and approach food. To create my food philosophy, I sat down one day and scribbled on a notepad what my beliefs were about good food. Then I used all the words I had written down and assembled them into positive statements in terms of my relationship with food. I went through several iterations of identifying the right words to define my values before creating the following food philosophy, which I use to guide my food choices.

I BELIEVE THAT FOOD SHOULD TASTE GOOD, NOURISH THE BODY AND PRESERVE HEALTH.

STICKING TO IT

Despite having a clear intention about the new, much healthier way I wanted to eat, changing my deeply rooted Southern eating habits was one of the hardest things I had ever done. I didn't have any family members to turn to for guidance about healthier ways to cook, and my friends couldn't help me, either. I found it incredibly frustrating to make a change when I felt like I was on an island with no hope of rescue.

But the longest journey begins with a single step, and the momentum I needed came from making one small change after another. I knew each step was bringing me closer to a healthier lifestyle. Although I was far from a complete lifestyle makeover, I could see that the goals I had set for myself were achievable, as long as I kept reaching for the finish line.

> "To wish to be well
> is a part of becoming well."
> **SENECA**

I didn't start my journey to better eating habits and more physical activity just to reach a particular pant size or to lose a specific number of pounds. I was attracted to eating better food because of the immense sense of empowerment I felt from being in control of my food choices and my health. Remember in Chapter 1, I mentioned you can tell if the changes you're making are working because you feel more pull toward good habits and less of a push away from them? Being in control of my food choices was empowering, and I'll discuss that in greater detail in Chapter 8. That feeling of empowerment can translate into feelings of pride and hope for a more vibrant future. I had never before considered my relationship with food as an expression of personal freedom or as a tool to inspire others. Prior to this point in my life, my power to eat right and care for my body in a nourishing way had yielded to old habits, family traditions, relationships with friends, fast-food restaurants, and food marketers.

Today, I'm 100 percent responsible for my food choices. But despite our best intentions, we all face days where situations arise that tempt us to compromise on our convictions.

Take stress. Like many people, I used to use food to deal with stress. I was fed up with my job as a high school biology teacher because I was underpaid and overworked. I was frustrated living in a tiny one-bedroom apartment situated beside noisy neighbors who were unrelenting insomniacs. On top of that, I was a full-time graduate student working on my master's degree in molecular biology. I was so busy just trying to keep up with the pace of work and school that I didn't take time to think about my diet, other than to recognize I needed to eat. At the time, what I ate didn't really matter. I was so busy *in* my life that I didn't have time to work *on* my life.

Although I had a full-time job, a loving family, several good friends, and a wonderful boyfriend, there was no excuse for neglecting to properly care for my body. Once I began to fully see the negative direction my health was headed, the thought of developing diabetes, cancer, or high blood pressure like other family members took up residence in my mind, persistently nudging me to change my course of action.

There are ways you, too, can avoid overeating when you're feeling emotional or stressed, and they're mostly related to what's going on inside your head. Your actions are a reflection of your thoughts. You've heard the saying, "What you think about, you bring about." Begin to think about the benefits of eating and living healthier. Consider the impact of the poor eating choice you're about to make on your short- and long-term health goals. Create or seek out positive affirmations that will help calm you during stressful times. Get in the habit of carrying around healthful snacks, such as nuts, string cheese, or whole-wheat crackers so you can reach for those when you're angry, tired, bored or anxious. Establish a ritual of taking a five-minute "time out" when you're feeling out of control. You can use those five minutes to go for a quick walk or engage in a deep-breathing exercise.

IT ISN'T TOO LATE

Anyone can eat themselves to death, but only a small percentage of people are able to make significant and lasting changes in their eating habits. In fact, statistics show of those who do successfully lose weight, 90 to 95 percent are unable to keep the weight off over the long term. Junk food, processed food, and fast-food marketers would have families believe that we don't have time to cook and that we can't afford to eat healthier food. This notion is far from the truth. With a little planning, a well-stocked pantry and refrigerator, and a core set of recipes that fit your family's taste and lifestyle, healthier meals are actually easier and more convenient than restaurant meals or processed foods.

Chopped nuts and fresh fruits, like apples and bananas, are delicious in their raw form and can be prepared in a matter of minutes. Studies show that kids and adults alike will reach for foods that are most readily available. If you have potato chips on the counter, that's what your spouse and kids will reach for. But, guess what? If you have freshly cut apple, strawberries, grapes, or cantaloupe in a bowl on the kitchen counter, *that's* the snack food they'll reach for! Most people naturally want to take the easy route, so if you have a ready-made and easily accessible snack on the kitchen counter, your kids won't pass it by to search the pantry or fridge for something they have to prepare for themselves. They just won't do it. Many times we say our kids are lazy. Well, this is an area where their laziness can actually be an asset!

QUICK WINS TIPS

Visit my blog, The Inspiring Cook—at www.tonyapeele.com/blog— for tips, tools and inspiration to help you and your family cook and eat more natural foods at home. Leave me a comment after each visit so I'll know you stopped by.

Once I learned to cook a few simple meals, got the hang of packing healthy snacks, and exercised consistently, I knew it was possible for me to change my habits. I believed that if I could transform my deeply rooted eating habits, my experience and knowledge would enable me to use my voice to help educate and empower family, friends and other women like me to take personal responsibility for their food choices and their health.

Adult and childhood obesity is growing at an alarming rate, and it can rip our families apart if we don't take action *right now!* Two-thirds of adults in this country are overweight or obese, and, sadly, one-third of children in America are overweight or obese. For adults and kids alike, those extra pounds greatly increase the risk of developing a range of chronic diseases that diminish—and in some cases, even extinguish—quality of life, including high blood pressure, heart disease, type 2 diabetes, and some cancers. In Chapter 4, you can take a closer look at the risks these diseases create for your future.

Inaction is no longer an option for American families. This generation of children—your children and mine—are the first not expected to outlive their parents. Do you know what this means? It means that if we don't start taking our eating habits seriously and make a concerted effort to clean up our diets, we may be going to our children's funerals!

If we love our families, we have to change. It's that simple. I encourage you to embrace the opportunity to commit yourself and your family to a healthful *life*.

One morning before work, I heard Alexandra Penney, a Bernie Madoff victim and author of *Lessons From Huge Loss,* speaking on *Good Morning America* about the wisdom she gained from her recent financial tragedy. Her advice to others: "Not to have lived to the fullest is the saddest, most irresponsible life I can think of." I share her quote with you to illustrate that it's not too late to take a different path—one that will lead you toward a life full of good health, mobility, joy, vitality, and longevity.

What you eat matters more than you think. You can change your lifestyle anytime you choose. And since you're a role model, you're empowered to help change the lives of your family as well. What's holding you back from deciding to eat and live better? Leaving your food life up to circumstance will only increase your odds of developing the lifestyle-related diseases I mentioned earlier.

Good food builds healthy bodies and minds and strong families. If you're ready to start living the healthiest and happiest life you possibly can, I encourage you to start here.

QUICK WINS TIPS

You *can* encourage your family to eat healthier. Here are a few pointers:

1. Ask your kids to help you plan and prepare a healthy family meal.

2. Make healthy snacks the easy choice. Make cut-up fruit, homemade fruit smoothies, whole grain crackers, nuts and bottled water readily available.

3. Repeatedly expose kids to fruit, vegetables, beans, nuts, and other nutritious foods – even if they didn't like them the first time.

4. Keep the foods that tempt you out of the house.

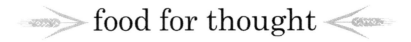

food for thought

- You can acquire the skills and tools to improve the way you and your family eat. It's never too late.

- Be mindful of the negative impact excessive eating out has on your family's health. It may seem like a smart move when you're short on time, but in the end, the health cost will outweigh the perceived benefit of a convenient meal.

- Our kids watch everything we do, even our poor eating habits. Let's be good role models.

- Don't dismiss home-cooked meals as a thing of the past! Eating at home helps you eat healthier, save money, and strengthen family bonds.

- While kids are young, teach them to grow, shop, cook, and eat nutritious whole foods.

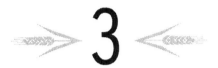

IS AMERICA'S CHOICE YOUR FAMILY'S CHOICE?

Most American families eat with a certain degree of carelessness, despite the fact that obesity, healthy diets, chronic illness, and weight loss are heavily discussed and sought-after topics in this country. Obesity concerns, stressful and demanding lifestyles, and a failing economy should force families to take a closer look at their eating habits. Nevertheless, kids and adults in this country are more overweight, out of shape and sickly than ever before.

Our fast-paced, convenience-driven lifestyle has transformed the way most families eat into a culture that's almost completely reliant upon highly refined carbohydrates, processed meats, and scarce amounts of fresh fruits and vegetables. The way most of America eats, commonly referred to as the Standard American Diet (SAD), has negative and far-reaching implications for the health of today's modern family. The diet of most American families is full of hydrogenated oil (transfat), high-fructose corn syrup, sodium nitrate and monosodium glutamate (MSG)—far from anything resembling a healthy diet.

> "One of the very nicest things about life
> is the way we must regularly stop whatever it is
> we are doing and devote our attention to eating."
> **LUCIANO PAVAROTTI, FROM *PAVAROTTI: MY OWN STORY***

Although it seems the odds are stacked against adopting lifestyle habits that are geared toward eating healthier, understanding the key trends that dictate the poor eating choices of most American families is your best weapon for successfully navigating your family toward better choices. For that reason, in Chapter 3, we'll take a close look at three choices many families make that greatly contribute to unhealthy eating, and we'll help you recognize if your family has also fallen into a trap of eating what's cheap, fast and convenient. In case you find your family needs to make some different choices, this chapter includes steps you can take *now* to get on the straight and narrow.

FOLLOWING THE HERD

None of us lives on an island. We are influenced by our environment and the habits of those closest to us more than we realize. So what one family member does has a huge impact on the habits and behaviors of other members of that family. In my natural food workshops, I often use the analogy of "herd behavior" to illustrate this point.

If you're not familiar with the concept of herd behavior, here's a quick explanation. Psychological and economic research has identified herd behavior in humans to explain the phenomenon of large numbers of people acting in the same way at the same time without planned action. Herd behavior is common during major events like stock market bubbles and street demonstrations, but it can also be seen in everyday decision-making, judgment, and opinion-forming, like whether to make a second trip to the buffet bar. My mom had a more practical way of explaining this behavior to my brother and me when we were growing up. When we were about to do something dumb just because one of our friends was doing it, she would ask us, "If everyone else jumps off a cliff, are you guys going to jump, too?" Each and every time she asked us that question it made us re-evaluate our actions and our ability to think for ourselves.

Years ago, when my diet included too much sugar, saturated fat, meat, and fried foods, I wasn't thinking for myself but was merely following my "herd." My family and friends ate this way, so I did, too. In my household, we ate a traditional Southern diet. Either chicken or beef was the focal point of the meal. Occasionally we had fish, but it was always fried. Vegetables—usually greens, potatoes, corn, beans, or cabbage—rounded out the meal. Vegetables were seasoned with butter, salt, and other seasonings. Meats were usually fried or baked. I never gave much thought to the immediate and long-term effects these habits could have on my health and the quality of my life. I was simply on autopilot.

Whenever I ate out, I tended to gravitate toward restaurants with a large buffet, like Golden Corral or Old Country Buffet because, after all, it was a better deal, right? I got in line just like everyone else and filled my plate as full as I could get it. Knowing how to pack a plate full of food without any spilling over on the buffet bar or the floor actually requires skill! And even though my first plate of food was enough to feed two people, I *always* went back for seconds. Second helpings were instinctive to me because I had learned from my herd that it was a waste of money to pay for a buffet and make only one trip to the bar.

IT'S YOUR CHOICE

Rates of overweight and obesity have increased dramatically in the United States over the past 30 years. This epidemic weight gain is due in large part to current eating trends that proliferate poor food choices. In many American households, poor food choices have become accepted as normal eating habits. Our busy, overextended lifestyles are rapidly eroding the fabric of our families. We don't have enough time to plan, shop, and prepare meals at home, so junk food and takeout prevails. And since we aren't cooking many meals at home, we aren't eating meals together at home. Family members are scattered in different directions, grabbing what they can find to eat along the way. There are few discussions around the dinner table, despite the fact that research shows that teens who eat with their families are 40 percent more likely to talk to their parents about problems.

I asked numerous families, as well as conducted research, about the top behaviors that drive unhealthy eating habits in busy families (which seems to be *all* families in America). The top culprits that get so many families off-track include eating away from home, consuming large portion sizes (obtained when dining out), and unhealthy snacking. When parents are busy, tired and stressed, they often rely on restaurant or takeout meals or excessive snack foods to tied their families over. Take a moment to reflect on your family's lifestyle. What choices are you making about family meals?

Choice No. 1: Eating Away From Home

A busy schedule, two working parents, kids, pets, and social obligations are a recipe for a restaurant meal. Hectic lifestyles lead a large number of U.S. households toward meals that are fast, affordable, and quick, which typically means they're consuming highly processed, high-fat and low-fiber foods.

Now more than ever before, American families are spending more money on food eaten away from home. Research shows that the consumption of food outside the home has increased since the mid-20th century, with the rate of spending rising from 34 percent of the food budget in 1970 to 47 percent in the late 1990s. This parallels the increase in number of food-service establishments, which has almost doubled from 491,000 in 1972 to 878,000 in 2004. In other words, families don't have to look far to find sit-down and fast-food restaurants, cafes, or street vendors for their daily sustenance.

Unfortunately, the trend of eating out has not only swept across American households but transformed the way families eat across the globe. Countries such as China and Japan are becoming "Americanized" through the integration of fast-food and convenience foods into everyday diets. Today there are more than 30,000 McDonald's outlets worldwide, and half of them are outside U.S. borders. The growth of fast-food restaurants is soaring in these countries, and their citizens are falling prey to the taste, convenience, and popularity of calorie-dense, nutrient-poor American meals.

QUICK WINS TIPS

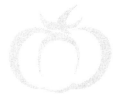

Plan, shop, and cook meals at home at least twice a week. Then gradually work your way up to cooking and eating at home at least four times per week.

Choice No. 2: Large Portion Sizes

One visible characteristic that makes restaurant dining so popular these days is the trend toward large portion sizes. Most sit-down and fast-food restaurants are able to provide consumers with a large amount of food for a very affordable price. Consumers view these offerings as a value and patronize establishments that offer a lot of food for their money. But when the health implications are considered, large portions don't look like such a good deal after all.

A number of factors contribute to the rising rates of adult and childhood obesity in this country, but the bottom line is we gain weight when we take in more calories than we burn. As I've stated before, when we gain weight, we put ourselves at risk for diet-related illnesses like high blood pressure, heart disease, type 2 diabetes, and cancer.

In many cases, we eat too much because we're offered too much. Our food portions have expanded so much that very few people actually know what a standard serving size is. A huge misconception is that a serving is equal to the amount served. In many cases, this is far from the truth. Consider the Grilled Salmon Burger from Red Robin restaurant, which comes on a whole grain bun with bistro sauce, red onions, tomatoes and lettuce. Sounds healthy, right? Salmon is rich in omega-3 fatty acids, which are touted for heart health. Whole grains are a good source of fiber. Red onions, tomatoes, and lettuce are vegetables. So this burger should seemingly get an automatic thumbs up, right? Not exactly. According to TheDailyPlate.com, a free online source of calorie counts and nutrition facts for more than 600,000 foods, one Grilled Salmon Burger contains 806 calories and 52 grams of carbohydrates. If you eat the fries that typically come with the burger, add another 390 calories. This one order will net you nearly 1,200 calories in one sitting—definitely not healthy!

A recent study published in the *American Journal of Public Health* confirmed that a huge discrepancy exists between standard USDA and FDA portion sizes and actual marketplace servings. According to the study's findings, the largest discrepancy occurred in the cookie category, with a 700 percent difference between measured and standard portion sizes. Other foods tested included cooked pasta, steaks and bagels, which exceeded standards by 480 percent, 224 percent, and 195 percent, respectively.

Thus, eating more meals away from home coupled with larger food portions has created a perfect storm for obesity and its related diseases. Not only do large food portions provide too many calories, but the nature of the food itself—often high-salt and high-sugar—encourages people to eat more. Studies even show that restaurants use carefully designed tactics to get consumers to eat more.

turning the tables

A 2010 CNN report on restaurants' table turnover tricks found that restaurateurs do any of the following to encourage you to eat more and faster:

- Play loud music to make customers eat faster and drink more.
- Seat customers in the middle of the restaurant, surrounded by chaos.
- Use uncomfortable chairs.
- Display dessert trays in customers' view.
- Decorate dining areas with warm colors like red, orange and yellow to stimulate the desire to eat.

QUICK WINS TIPS

Compensate for eating larger portions at one meal by eating fewer calories during the rest of the day. You could also eat half your meal at one sitting and save the rest for later.

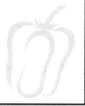

What do we typically do after consuming such large amounts of food? We sit. According to the National Center for Health Statistics' *2008 Chartbook on Trends in the Health of Americans*, only 30 percent of the U.S. population engages in regular leisure-time physical activity. There's no question: The way we eat and our inactive lifestyles weigh heavily on the growing trend toward overweight and obesity.

Choice No. 3: Unhealthy Snacking

Americans do a lot of snacking. According to a national consumer survey by Simmons Market Research Bureau, 25 percent of adults snack between meals. Wouldn't it be great if all that snacking was done sensibly? But the truth is, snacking isn't something we do well in this country.

One unhealthy habit that drives so many people to reach for snacks is lack of meal preparation. According to a recent survey conducted by the American Institute for Cancer Research (AICR), 1 in 8 Americans is skipping meals more often. According to recent surveys from market research firm Packaged Facts and The Calorie Control Council, an international association representing low-calorie and reduced-fat food and beverage manufacturers, 33 percent of Americans skip meals and graze on snack foods when they're on the go. And that's not all: The rate has increased significantly since 2004! Respondents stated lack of free time to prepare healthy, nutritious meals as the major factor that drives frequent snacking, totaling about 20 percent of their daily calories.

Unhealthy snacking wreaks havoc on your body and sets you up for a cycle of unhealthy eating. The most popular snack foods are carbohydrates—the refined kind—mainly chips, cookies, crackers, sodas, candy, and the like. These foods cause spikes in blood sugar, making you feel jittery, unfocused, and lethargic. Once your blood sugar dips, you'll feel cravings again, coupled with low energy. These bodily signals will send you running back for more food. You again reach for a carbohydrate-rich meal, such as fast food, and the cycle starts all over again. By the end of the day you've consumed way more calories than you can burn off.

Done responsibly, snacking can be part of a healthy diet. Eating a healthy snack is a great way to add more nourishing foods to your diet, like fruits and vegetables, plus snacks help you tame your hunger so you can eat sensibly at meal time. In fact, you should rely on snacks for at least two of your daily meals.

To keep your metabolism revved up, your mood stable, and your brain functioning at high capacity, experts recommend eating five to six small meals in place of three large meals. Most people are accustomed to eating three big meals each day, so you'll have to make a conscious effort to plan and eat smaller meals throughout your day. Let's clarify: Snacks aren't meals, so aim for healthy snacks that are no more than 200 or 250 total calories.

The population most at risk from poor snacking habits is our children. A recent study published in the journal *Health Affairs* found that frequent snacking accounts for more than 27 percent of most kids' daily calorie intake. The largest increase in snacking was seen in young kids ages 2 to 6, who consumed more than 182 calories each day from snacks.

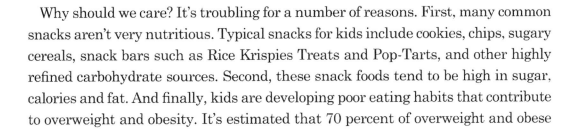

QUICK WINS TIPS

- Offer your kids snacks on fun plates. Plates of different shapes, sizes and colors are appealing to younger kids.

- Use colorful plastic forks and spoons.

- Serve water in glasses with neon straws.

Why should we care? It's troubling for a number of reasons. First, many common snacks aren't very nutritious. Typical snacks for kids include cookies, chips, sugary cereals, snack bars such as Rice Krispies Treats and Pop-Tarts, and other highly refined carbohydrate sources. Second, these snack foods tend to be high in sugar, calories and fat. And finally, kids are developing poor eating habits that contribute to overweight and obesity. It's estimated that 70 percent of overweight and obese kids will become overweight and obese adults. And weight gain isn't the only problem: Unhealthy snacking also increases risk for dental problems, such as cavities.

IMPACT ON LEARNING AND BEHAVIOR

Children have small stomachs that don't hold much food at one time, so those little tummies need to be refilled regularly. Smart snacks can contribute to children's overall nutritional well-being if they provide quality nutrition for good health and normal growth.

Kids eat snacks at school, at home, in the car, and practically everywhere they go. Make sure the snacks they eat are healthful by preparing and packaging them at home. Zip-lock bags and storage containers make transporting snacks to and from school easy. When your family is out and about, be sure to pack a lunch tote or small cooler with plenty of healthy beverages and snacks. This will ensure healthy options are available when your family gets hungry and will reduce your reliance on unhealthy convenience or fast foods.

QUICK WINS TIPS

- Select snack foods that satisfy hunger, supply the body with energy, and provide quality nutrients.

- Have tasty and nutritious snacks available for your kids to enjoy. Always strive to make the healthy choice the easy choice.

- Make snacks a part of your family's healthy diet by structuring snacks on a schedule.

THERE'S NO EXCUSE

Personal responsibility plays a huge role in your quality of health, but you can't ignore societal factors—such as education level, income, and the condition of the neighborhood environment—that have a great impact on your ability to make good food choices and, ultimately, manage your health. Although not everyone has access to the highest-quality food, each of us is empowered to make small, simple changes in our food choices that will have some measure of positive effect on our health. Remember our mantra: *Small changes matter and can lead to Quick Wins for your health.*

HEALTHY SNACKS

The Center for Science in the Public Interest, a consumer advocate for nutrition and health, food safety, and food alcohol policy, has useful guides on healthy snacks for home and on the go. Here are a few suggestions from its *Healthy School Snacks Guide*.

Fruits: Whole, Sliced, Cubed, Canned, Frozen, or Dried

Apples	Apricots	Bananas	Blackberries
Blueberries	Cantaloupe	Cherries	Grapefruit
Grapes	Honeydew Melon	Kiwis	Mandarin Oranges
Mangoes	Nectarines	Oranges	Peaches
Pears	Pineapple	Plums	Raspberries
Strawberries	Tangerines	Watermelon	Applesauce

Note: Ensure fruit cups and canned fruit are purchased in water, 100% fruit juice, or light syrup.

Vegetables: Whole, Sliced, Cubed, or Dried

Broccoli	Baby Carrots	Cauliflower	Celery Sticks
Cucumbers	Red Peppers	Green Peppers	Snap Peas
Snow Peas	String Beans	Cherry Tomatoes	Squash Slices
Zucchini Slices			

Whole Grains (100% Whole Wheat)

Pitas	English Muffins	Tortillas	Breakfast cereal
Crackers	Rice Cakes	Popcorn	Granola
Cereal Bars	Pretzels	Breadsticks	

Low-Fat Dairy

Natural cheese	Milk	Cottage Cheese	Eggs
Yogurt	Cream Cheese	Homemade Smoothies	

Beverages

Water	100% Fruit Juice	Soy and Rice Drinks	Seltzer

Quick Wins are achievable, irrespective of your socio-economic status. Repeating your actions consistently and systematically will provide the momentum you need to steer your family away from obesity-related illnesses. In the next chapter, we'll tackle the four big health risks that could greatly impact your family's future if you don't make small changes *now* in the way you eat.

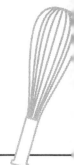

BELIEVE IT OR NOT
One slice of Sbarro's Stuffed Pepperoni Pizza contains 960 calories, 42g fat and 3,200mg sodium.

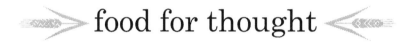

food for thought

- The Standard American Diet, rich in highly refined carbohydrates and processed meats but low on fruits and vegetables, doesn't have to be the norm for your family.

- Cooking and eating dinner together at home instills the value of good nutrition and family togetherness.

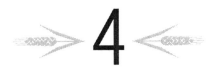

THE BIG FOUR RISKS FOR THE FUTURE

Now that you have a good idea how the major lifestyle choices many Americans make lead to poor eating habits, let's delve into the negative impact those poor choices can have on your health and quality of life. It's no doubt that the Standard American Diet (SAD), characterized by high-fat, high-salt, and highly processed foods, is taking a toll on our youth and adult populations. It's pretty difficult to live a healthy and happy life when so many of us are suffering from, or at risk of, serious obesity-related illnesses. If you aren't suffering from a chronic illness yourself, chances are great you have a close family member or friend who is.

The United States isn't alone when it comes to soaring rates of obesity-related disease. In fact, the World Health Organization (WHO) stated in a 2000 report that obesity has become a global problem. As global rates of obesity have increased over the past decade, so has the global prevalence of high blood pressure, heart disease, Type 2 diabetes, and some cancers. Once considered a problem only in higher-income countries, escalating overweight and obesity rates are now affecting low- and middle-income countries. To address the global impact of obesity, WHO has named obesity as one of the greatest health problems facing the world today. Our personal success and the prosperity of our nation have led to societal and behavioral patterns that revolve around calorie-dense diets and sedentary lifestyles. Despite the profound changes taking place around us to increase urbanization and industrialization and minimize traditional lifestyles, each of us still retains control to make the right choices for our health. Your next preventive step is to arm yourself with the knowledge you need to take action.

This includes calculating your body mass index (and that of each of your family members), measuring waist circumference, and identifying any risk factors you may have for developing one of the four major chronic lifestyle diseases. In this chapter, we'll discuss what you can do to reduce the risk of developing high blood pressure, heart disease, type 2 diabetes, or cancer that could be knocking at your family's door.

FIGHTING BACK

To help you further understand the connection between food and health, let's explore some of the risks involved with poor eating habits. Unhealthy lifestyle habits continue to contribute to the majority of illness and death in the United States every year. Rates of adult obesity in the United States have doubled since 1985 and continue to rise. A 2009 study led by Dr. Ken Thorpe, an Emory University health-care economist, found that if obesity continues at its present rate, 43 percent of Americans will be obese by 2018, costing the health-care system $344 billion annually.

An alarming 69 percent of overweight people report having been stigmatized by their doctors, with patients reporting that medical professionals are dismissing their health concerns by attributing their weight issues to lack of willpower. As a result, overweight patients are reluctant to seek medical care and cancel or delay medical appointments and preventative health-care services.

Stigma, bias and discrimination against overweight and obese people are wrong. All people deserve to have their basic human rights protected. Treating people unfairly does nothing to help them gain the knowledge and confidence to make different and better choices for themselves.

More healthful diets and increased physical activity would reduce illnesses associated with obesity and subsequently help to reduce the long-term medical costs that are being driven up by obesity-related diseases.

Studies show that poor nutrition and lack of physical activity are associated with 300,000 deaths each year in the United States. High blood pressure, heart disease, type 2 (adult-onset) diabetes and some cancers—what I call "The Big Four"—have been described in medical and consumer literature as being largely preventable.

What does this mean for you? It means that if you adopt a more nourishing diet and exercise regularly, chances are good that you can avoid The Big Four. How empowering is that! So even if any of The Big Four run in your family, you can prevent or delay the onset of these diseases by switching to a diet rich in fruits, vegetables, whole grains, legumes (beans), and other nutrient-dense foods that have been shown to help the body function properly.

weight matters

In some literature, you may see The Big Four referred to as obesity-related diseases. The term refers to any disease for which obesity is a significant risk factor and includes a large number of diseases, including:

- Type 2 diabetes
- High blood pressure
- Stroke
- Heart failure
- Cancer (certain forms, such as prostate, colon and rectum)
- Gallstones and gall bladder disease
- Gout and gouty arthritis
- Osteoarthritis (of the knees, hips, and lower back)
- Sleep apnea
- Pickwickian syndrome (red face, under-ventilation and drowsiness)

Source: MedicineNet.com

WHAT IS OBESITY?

If you want to tackle The Big Four, we need to start at the beginning. How can you tell if you're overweight, or obese? It's actually quite simple. The body mass index (BMI) is the medical standard used to determine if adults are at a healthy weight, overweight or obese. BMI is estimated by a crude calculation based on a person's weight and height. You calculate BMI by dividing weight in pounds (lbs) by height in inches (in) squared and multiplying by a conversion factor of 703. Here's what the formula looks like:

BMI = (Weight in pounds) / (Height in inches x Height in inches) x 703

Now, let's plug in some numbers: **Your weight =** 150 lbs; **height** = 5'5" (65 inches), so your BMI would be: (150 ÷ [65 x 65]) x 703 = 24.96.

There are also many websites that will automatically calculate your BMI for you. WebMD.com, for instance, has an excellent, user-friendly BMI calculator on its website (www.webmd.com/diet/calc-bmi-plus).

Although BMI isn't a direct measure of body fat, it is recognized as a more accurate indicator of overweight and obesity than weight measurements alone. According to WHO's International BMI Classification, for adults (the standards are the same for men and women), a BMI value under 18.5 is considered underweight, values 18.5 to 24.9 are considered normal and 25 to 29 is considered overweight. Obesity is defined as having a BMI of 30 or greater.

Since there's currently no global standard definition of childhood obesity, the BMI isn't used to measure overweight and obesity in children aged 5 to 19 years. To measure obesity in children or teenagers, a percentile of BMI is used. A BMI for age is plotted on gender-specific growth charts developed by the Centers for Disease Control (CDC) and indicates a child's BMI in relation to that of other children. Keep a record of you and your child's BMI in your "Quick Wins Health Journal" (see Appendix A), along with your blood pressure, cholesterol number, and other important personal medical information.

BMI WEIGHT STATUS

Below 18.5 » Underweight

18.5 - 24.9 » Normal

25.0 - 29.9 » Overweight

30.0 and Above » Obese

Although your BMI may be the same as someone else's, the distribution of your body fat could be different and impact your risk for developing one of The Big Four diseases. If you carry excess body fat primarily around your waist (i.e., pear-shaped), you're at greater risk for chronic obesity-related health conditions. If your body fat is evenly distributed, then your risk of these diseases is lower. The WHO waist-circumference criteria recommend that women aim for a waist circumference of less than 35 inches. The limit for male waistlines is 40 inches. Just like calculating your BMI, figuring out your waistline size is easy to do. A simple sewing tape measure will give you an idea of your waist size.

"He who has health, has hope; and
he who has hope, has everything."
ARABIAN PROVERB

If your waist measures larger than it should for optimal health or your BMI falls within the overweight or obese category, stay calm. This book provides you with practical approaches for building achievable changes into your eating style that can help you decrease your body fat and reduce your odds of developing The Big Four.

THE BIG FOUR

In the following sections, we'll discuss The Big Four one by one to ensure you know what they are, the impact they can have your health, and most important, what you can do *right now* to make lifelong changes that will keep you and your family healthy.

High Blood Pressure

My stepfather had a stroke resulting from unmanaged high blood pressure in January 1996 during a huge North Carolina snow storm. He was a relatively young man of 40 at the time. High blood pressure (hypertension) is the leading cause, as well as the most controllable risk factor, of stroke, and it currently affects about 50 million (or 1 in 4) American adults. More than any other race, African Americans have the highest risk of high blood pressure, with 35 percent of the population being affected, according to the CDC. The death rate from this disease is 20 percent among this demographic, which is twice the percentage of that among white Americans.

Blood pressure is a measurement of the force of blood pushing against blood-vessel walls. It's normal for blood pressure to rise and fall, but when blood is restricted from flowing freely through the vessels, the force of blood increases, resulting in an elevation of blood pressure. Increased blood pressure for prolonged periods of time is particularly dangerous because it forces the heart to work harder.

My stepfather was diagnosed with high blood pressure long before his stroke occurred, but he had stopped taking his prescribed medications to control his blood pressure. He also wasn't seeing his doctor regularly to monitor his disease. Hypertension is known as the "silent killer" because it can damage the body without causing any symptoms. Regular doctor visits are vital for people at risk or suffering from hypertension.

One day my stepfather started feeling a little odd and finally decided to go in for a checkup. When he arrived at the doctor's office, his blood pressure was so high that his doctor wanted to immediately admit him into the hospital, but my stepfather refused hospitalization. At home later that evening, he began to suffer from the early stages of a stroke.

common warning signs of stroke

If you experience any of these warning signs, seek medical attention immediately.

- Sudden numbness or weakness in the face, arm or leg (usually on just one side of the body)
- Sudden confusion, trouble speaking or understanding
- Sudden trouble seeing in one or both eyes
- Sudden trouble walking, dizziness, loss of balance or coordination
- Headache

Source: American Stroke Association and Mayo Clinic

A stroke happens when blood flow is restricted to a part of the brain. This can occur when a blood vessel in the brain is blocked or bursts. My stepfather spent the next eight days in a Virginia hospital trauma unit. The impact of a stroke can leave a person with visible physical impairments, such as weakness on one side of the body. Fortunately, my stepfather's stroke didn't leave him physically impaired (i.e., left or right side paralysis). However, our family soon learned of the significant impact the stroke did have on his cognitive abilities. For example, drinking a glass of water proved too difficult for him. He could recognize a glass of water and could pick it up, but would then simply release the glass from his hands when he was done drinking. The glass fell to his bed and water went everywhere. His team of doctors explained that his brain couldn't send his hand a signal to put the glass back on the tray, so he simply dropped it.

I recall his inability to do simple things like write his name, tell time, count from 1 to 10, get dressed or eat with utensils. This lasted for days and even months after his stroke. He spent the next 12 months, maybe longer, in home therapy with staff that helped him to retrain his brain to coordinate basic everyday functions. All in all, it took about three years for my stepfather to reclaim his independence and perform the simple activities of daily living that many of us take for granted.

The controllable risk factors for high blood pressure include obesity (BMI ≥ 30.0), high-salt diets, alcohol use, inactivity and stress. A study published in the *Journal of the American Heart Association* showed that a low-risk lifestyle was associated with a reduced risk of multiple chronic diseases and may be beneficial in the prevention of stroke.

The DASH (Dietary Approaches to Stop Hypertension) Diet and the Mediterranean Diet, rich in fruits, vegetables, whole grains, and low-fat dairy, in conjunction with reduced sodium intake, can lower blood pressure significantly. Visit the American Stroke Association (www.strokeassociation.org) for information. Many people believe the myth that hypertension is a normal part of aging. On the contrary, hypertension is *not* a part of healthy aging—and *can* be prevented.

QUICK WINS TIPS

- Avoid processed foods and fast foods. Fresh is best!

- Prepare more home-cooked meals so you can control salt content.

- Read food labels to determine sodium content in packaged foods. Remember, salt can be added in many forms and included on ingredients labels as baking powder, celery salt, garlic salt, monosodium glutamate (MSG), rock salt, sea salt, sodium, sodium bicarbonate, or sodium nitrate/nitrite.

- Buy low-sodium foods.

- Think of the food you eat as medicine. Begin to explore foods that offer rich, natural sources of fiber, vitamins, minerals and antioxidants. These foods have the power of health.

Heart Disease

Heart disease has been declared the number-one killer of men and women in the United States, resulting in over 600,000 deaths each year. Obesity is now recognized as a major risk factor for heart disease, which can lead to heart attack. So as the rate of obesity continues to climb in adult and youth populations, the incidence of heart disease in this country is also expected to increase. In addition to obesity, several other risk factors also play a role in the development of heart disease. These risk factors are probably familiar to you. They include smoking, diabetes, high blood pressure, increasing age and abnormal cholesterol levels.

Even if you have no other risk factors, obesity alone can dramatically increase your risk for heart disease. But generally speaking, most people engage in more than one of the unhealthy behaviors mentioned above. According to the AHA, obesity negatively impacts heart health by:

- Raising blood cholesterol and triglyceride levels
- Lowering HDL, or "healthy" cholesterol
- Raising blood pressure
- Increasing the risk for diabetes

Since diet plays such a key role in weight management, it stands to reason that if your family takes steps to eat healthier right now, you can clean up your diet, get your weight within a healthy range, and reduce your risk for heart disease. Start your fight against heart disease by incorporating one simple, healthful habit at a time.

You can begin by choosing to eat more whole grains—which contain fiber to help you feel full—over their highly refined counterparts like white bread. Another simple change you can incorporate is to stop using white rice and eat whole-grain brown rice instead. You can slowly acclimate your family to the taste and texture of brown rice by starting with a blend of half white rice and half brown rice, then gradually work your way up to all brown rice.

> Don't dig your grave with
> your own knife and fork.
> **ENGLISH PROVERB**

The AHA endorses a healthy diet of nutrient-dense foods full of vitamins, minerals, and fiber. Since physical inactivity is also a major risk factor for heart disease, the AHA recommends at least 30 minutes of moderate physical activity on most days of the week for adults 18 to 65. Children aged 2 and older should also engage in 30 minutes of age-appropriate physical activity daily.

The Mediterranean Diet, a heart-healthy eating style (not actually a diet) is endorsed by the AHA and embraces whole grains and other nutritious whole foods. The Mediterranean Diet incorporates the basics of healthy eating, plus flavorful, monounsaturated olive oil and red wine (optional). I prepare and eat Mediterranean-style foods often in my own kitchen and have personally found the food to be sensible, simple, avorful, and nutritious. Appendix E has great resources if you're interested in learning more about Mediterranean cuisine.

QUICK WINS TIPS

○ Learn how to eat for a healthy heart. Search "heart-healthy foods" online and make a list of at least one new food to add to your diet each week.

○ Purchase a copy of the American Heart Association's *Meals in Minutes* cookbook, which is chock-full of heart-healthy meals you and your family can prepare quickly and easily in minutes.

Type 2 Diabetes

Earlier this year, my mom's doctor expressed concern about her blood sugar. Her sugar levels weren't quite in the range for diabetes, but they were approaching a level of concern. Her doctor scheduled her for a fasting blood-glucose test for further diagnosis. Fasting blood-sugar tests measure blood glucose after you've fasted, or not eaten, for at least eight hours. It's often the first test performed to check for pre-diabetes and diabetes. Thankfully, mom was not diagnosed with full-blown diabetes, but she is considered "pre-diabetic," meaning she is at risk for developing diabetes if she doesn't take immediate and aggressive steps to manage her blood sugar.

As a first course of action, her doctor recommended she lose a few pounds and monitor her blood sugar regularly with a glucose monitor. Similar to the controllable risk factors for high blood pressure and heart disease, the primary risk factor for type 2 diabetes is obesity.

According to the American Dietetic Association, type 2 diabetes is the most common form of diabetes. In people with type 2 diabetes, their bodies don't produce enough insulin or their cells aren't able to recognize the insulin their body produces. A person with a genetic predisposition for diabetes and living a Western lifestyle (poor diet and sedentary lifestyle) is at greatest risk for developing type 2 diabetes. However, research shows that people living outside the Western influence of high-fat, high-salt, high-sugar, and heavily processed foods tend not to get type 2 diabetes, no matter how high their genetic risk.

Millions of people—23.6 million, or 7.8 percent of the population—in this country have been diagnosed with type 2 diabetes. Many others have the disease or are at significant risk for diabetes but don't know it.

The rise in obesity has led to dramatic increases over the past 20 years in the prevalence of type 2 diabetes in children and adolescents. As obesity rates continue to increase in these young populations, their risk of significant health consequences in the future dramatically escalates. The ultimate cost could be a shorter life. The impact of a chronic disease like diabetes in children is manifested by the extended period of time in which the body is battered by poor glucose regulation. For example, the eyes and kidneys of adults who become diabetic in their late 40s are potentially affected less by glucose irregulation than are the organs of young children who've been diagnosed in their early teens. Research shows that the longer people have diabetes, the more likely they are to develop devastating complications from the disease. Therefore, the impact of type 2 diabetes in youth populations is significant. What does all this mean for you? It means that although you may have genetic risk factors, it's possible to delay or even prevent the onset of diabetes. Remain focused on your healthy-eating goals. You really do have everything you need to adopt healthier lifestyle choices that will put good health within your reach.

QUICK WINS TIPS

° Focus more of your efforts on the prevention of diabetes in your home by adopting a healthy eating plan to keep your blood sugar under control. This includes eating small meals on a regular schedule, with a variety of fiber-rich fruits, vegetables and whole grains.

° Ask your doctor if you or your children are at risk for the disease.

Cancer

You may have noticed that poor eating habits and sedentary living are significant risk factors for high blood pressure, heart disease, and diabetes. The risks for cancer are no different. Each year, about 563,000 Americans die of cancer, and one-third of these deaths are linked to poor diet, physical inactivity and excess body weight.

Obesity fuels cancers of the breast, colon, esophagus, kidney and uterus, as well as other cancers that are driven by hormones like estrogen and insulin. The National Cancer Institute reports that obesity and physical inactivity may account for as much as 25 to 30 percent of these major cancers. Experts recommend preventing weight gain to reduce the risk of cancer. However, losing as little as 5 to 10 percent of your total weight is effective at reducing cancer risks.

I know the devastating impact of cancer on a family. In 2008, I lost my maternal grandmother to bone cancer. It was painful to watch the disease ravage her body and eventually steal her soul. Not only was she my grandmother, but she was one of my very best friends. I talked to her about every significant event in my life. When I was in my teens, I got so frustrated with my parents and their strict rules that I decided to run away from home. While my parents were at work, I packed my suitcase full of clothes, wrote my parents a goodbye note, and called my grandmother to pick me up. My plan was to "run away" to her house until my mom and dad decided to become more reasonable parents. As a parent now myself, I can only imagine how my parents must have laughed when they read my ridiculous note.

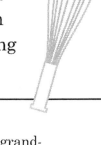

BELIEVE IT OR NOT
Chronic diseases are among the most common and costly health problems, but they're also among the most preventable diseases.

My grandma held a special place in the life of each of her children and grandchildren. She was so easy to talk with and so wise. As a result, she knew about every family member's "stuff." Good thing she never decided to blackmail any of us! Grandma was the glue that held our family together. Now that she's gone, her special ability to hold the family together is evident more now than ever.

Before my grandmother died, she had buried four of her sisters and brothers, who had also died from cancer.

YOUR CHALLENGE

To reduce your cancer risk, maintain a healthy body weight, eat a plant-based diet, exercise regularly, and avoid smoking. I challenge you to make eating healthier and exercising regularly a priority in your life.

Let's start with your diet. Do you know there are natural chemicals within whole foods that help the body repair and maintain itself? These plant chemicals, called phytonutrients, exist in a variety of fruits and vegetables and have antioxidant properties. Antioxidants are substances that fight free-radical damage. When cells use oxygen to carry out cellular functions, free radicals are produced as byproducts. These substances then move about the body, causing cellular damage. Antioxidants prevent and repair damage caused by free-radicals. Examples of common antioxidants include vitamins A, C and E; selenium, coenzyme Q10 (CoQ10), and glutathione. Other nutritive substances like indole-3-carbinol, lutein, bioflavonoids and resveratrol are also highly protective against cancer. By eating a variety of richly colored fruits, vegetables, beans and grains, you are assured of an ample supply of antioxidants into your diet.

Moving on to exercise, what should you do to lose unwanted pounds and reduce your risk of cancer? You must make healthier food choices and increase your physical activity. You already know that, right? But you probably want to know *how* to get started. Begin by reducing portion sizes of high-calorie foods, limit sugary beverages, and eat a rainbow of fruits and vegetables each day.

QUICK WINS TIPS

Schedule trips to the farmer's market and morning exercise times on your calendar just like you do with PTO meetings and dentist appointments. Why do you schedule these types of important appointments? So you won't forget them. That's the same approach you need to take to make sure you keep your appointments for healthy-living activities. Otherwise, you'll get so caught up in the daily grind that you won't make time to shop for nutritious fresh foods or to exercise daily. If you don't view these activities as essential appointments, they'll fall by the wayside.

If you're not exercising regularly, start by walking for 15 minutes a day. This is enough exercise to get you feeling better, but you have to work toward exercising a little bit more. The latest recommendations for adults call for at least 30 minutes of intentional moderate to vigorous activity a day. If you started with 15 minutes or less, you can work your way up to 30 minutes or more in no time at all. Try adding five extra minutes to your walk each day for a week until you reach your desired exercise goal.

According to the Physical Activity Guidelines for Americans, children aged 6 to 17 should get 60 minutes of physical activity daily. The guidelines state that adults need at least 2½ hours of moderate-intensity aerobic activity (e.g., brisk walking) every week and two or more days per week of muscle-strengthening activities that work all major muscle groups (legs, hips, back, abdomen, chest, shoulders and arms). There are no hard-and-fast rules for how you get your exercise, so be creative and let a physical family activity double as your exercise for the day. A game of soccer or tag with your kids and spouse in the backyard is great fun and can really get your heart pumping.

YOUR FUTURE BEGINS NOW

As you can see, changes in lifestyle, specifically healthier eating habits, regular physical activity, and maintaining optimal body weight, are highly effective in preventing The Big Four. Your healthy future awaits you. Make the ultimate choice to create the healthy future you deserve.

tonya's top 5

In addition to preventing The Big Four, there are other healthful reasons to eat a more nutritious diet. Here are my top five reasons for sticking with a healthy diet. Create your own reasons for eating better and begin to change your life today.

1. Maintain abundant energy.
2. Gain mental clarity and focus.
3. Avoid disease.
4. Look good.
5. Feel healthy and strong.

You can be a leader in creating and sustaining simple changes in your life that will make your whole family stronger. Begin by embracing one healthy change at a time until you gain momentum. Perhaps you can make the switch from white bread to whole-wheat bread. Another simple, but impactful, change you could make right now is to make water the preferred beverage at dinner time in your household. Purchase a sink drinking-water filter and keep your refrigerator stocked with reusable water containers that make it easy for your family to grab one when they're thirsty. In our house, each person has their own special water bottle, but you can always add initials or color coding with a permanent marker to designate each person's bottle.

As a role model for healthy habits, you'll inspire your loved ones to re-evaluate their lifestyle habits. As you change old habits and begin supporting your family along their journey, you'll strengthen your confidence and your family's commitment to a healthier diet.

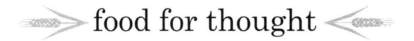

food for thought

○ Proper nutrition is a major key to long-lasting optimal health.

○ Know your health numbers (weight, waist circumference, blood pressure, blood glucose), and keep them in check. Record these values for each family member.

○ Chronic disease isn't a normal part of living.

○ Be proactive about your health—you have the power to create lifestyle change.

EMPOWER YOUR KIDS—AND FIGHT CHILDHOOD OBESITY

Our great-grandmothers would be appalled at the way most of us feed our children today. Many families rely so heavily on the convenience of fast food, packaged food, and highly processed food that it has transformed the way most children eat into a pattern that would be unrecognizable to our great-grandparents. As a result, our children are becoming overweight, obese, and unhealthy.

When I was growing up, things were much different. My mom prepared breakfast, lunch (on the weekends), and dinner for my brother and me almost every day. The exception was usually on Sundays, when we ate dinner at my grandma's house along with my mom's sisters, her brother, and their children. Eating out was an occasional treat for us. Once a month, my mom drove my brother and me to the State Employees Credit Union nearly 50 miles from our home where she deposited her paycheck. After that, we always went to Wendy's for a burger and fries. That's the one time of the month I remember eating out.

> **QUICK WINS TIPS**
>
> The healthiest meal is a home-cooked meal.

Today, this is the exception rather than the norm. More moms today, approximately 60 percent, work outside the home, leaving little time to cook for their families. Thus, eating out has become an integral part of our busy lifestyles. No wonder so many kids today are overweight. Experts have found that kids who eat meals outside the home tend to consume more food in general and more fried foods in particular, a significant contributor to weight gain.

In this chapter, we'll look at how much our lifestyle and our eating habits have changed in one generation, making many families reliant on fast and processed foods for nourishment. We'll also take a close look at the transformation families have gone through and its impact on our health and our children's ability to perform well in school. So prepare to arm yourself with even more steps you can take now to help kids eat healthier, be active, and learn better.

AIN'T NOTHIN' LIKE THE REAL THING

Parents have been led to believe that processed "food," like Fruit Roll-Ups and fruit leather, is just as good as the real thing. In case you're wondering what the difference is, fruit that's as flat and long as a ruler is considered "processed stuff" and a whole pear that's fresh, frozen or canned is the "real thing." While consumers continue to buy into the marketing notion of processed over real, families spend less and less time in the kitchen planning, cooking and eating healthy meals so they can make time for other activities. Yet our quest for quick fixes to solve our mealtime woes have gotten us nowhere in terms of our health.

QUICK WINS TIPS

To reduce the amount of chemicals you put into your body, decrease your use of packaged and processed foods. If you have to rely on them, check the nutrition labels and select those with the fewest additives.

Take, for example, some of the popular foods that many kids and adults consider a source of fruit. General Mills' Fruit by the Foot and Fruit Gushers are branded as fruit snacks and have become all the rage with kids. Through clever marketing, including bright colors, fun-looking characters, and an affordable price, these highly processed products have found their way into lunchboxes and pantries across the country.

Parents use fruit snacks as quick, convenient and affordable alternatives to real fresh fruit. When you have the choice of grabbing a "fruit" from the pantry vs. washing, peeling and cutting fresh fruit, the easier option usually wins. Yes, there are precut, prepackaged fruits like apples and carrots in the produce aisle, but they lose their muster rather quickly when parents have to contend with the cost of these healthier alternatives and the need for refrigeration. Heck, you can keep a fruit leather in your purse or your car for a month or more and just whip it out when the next snack attack strikes.

informed eating

Let's examine the nutrition facts label for Fruit by the Foot (see below). If parents read the nutrition label at all, they usually look for the number of calories and sometimes the amount of fat. Another key part of the label to consider is the list of ingredients. This tells you exactly what's in the food you're about to eat yourself or feed to your family.

The ingredients listed on the nutrition label are arranged from the greatest quantity to least. The less processed a food item is, the shorter the list will be. So the first five items on the list make up the majority of ingredients in the product. Typically, the healthiest products have ingredients you can pronounce. The second ingredient in Fruit by the Foot is added sugar. The third ingredient is maltodextrin, which is a common food additive. And the next ingredients are corn syrup (more sugar) and partially hydrogenated oil (trans fat).

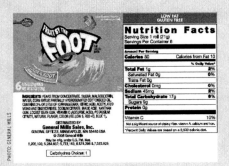

I know we're focusing on the first five ingredients, but I want you to continue scanning the remaining items in the list to see the other food additives and preservatives that make up this kid snack. Not all food additives and preservatives are harmful, but some of may be. The key is to know what you and your family are eating and to make an informed decision about whether you want to consume it or not.

Now tell me, would your great-grandmother recognize 12 inches of pear concentrate, sugar, and about 18 other ingredients rolled up and tucked into a foil-like package, like a piece of gum? Mine sure wouldn't. I can hear my great-grandmother's voice in my head now, saying, "Why not just give the child a pear?"

THE NEW NORM

It's amazing how much children's lifestyles have changed in just one generation. Unlike our parents' generation, we've become accustomed to fake foods that are full of refined sugars, salt, hydrogenated oil (trans fat), processed meats, and food additives like monosodium glutamate (MSG), aspartame, and artificial colors. When I say the word "fake," perhaps images of deeply hued plastic apples and oranges found in preschool kitchen play centers come to mind. Actually, what's being passed off as food today may not be far from that. But "fake food" refers to highly processed, highly refined boxed and restaurant food containing parts of foods, chemicals and preservatives. Fake food is basically devoid of nutritional value.

Examples of fake/highly processed food include lunch meats, potato chips, microwaveable noodles, and Rice Krispie treats. The original, unprocessed counterparts of these items have been stripped of minerals, vitamins, and fiber in order to make them quick and convenient. You may have some of these foods in your pantry or refrigerator. If so, you can find simple tips in Appendix D for converting the items in your pantry into more healthful alternatives.

> "As for butter versus margarine,
> I trust cows more than chemists."
> **JOAN GUSSOW**

Food manufacturers have responded rapidly to our growing impatience with food preparation in our kitchens, restaurants, and workplaces. We don't have a lot of time to spend "fussing" with food. We want to eat as soon as our brains get the first signal of hunger, we want food that tastes good, and we don't want to pay a lot for it. Our modern food expectations have birthed a multibillion-dollar industry of great-tasting, inexpensive, widely available, nutrient-poor convenience foods. Sadly, this poor eating trend, along with obesity, has become America's new "normal."

In fact, I recently heard a National Public Radio interview stating that the image of an undernourished child is no longer the emaciated child in Africa but the overweight child in this country. How can a significantly overweight child be undernourished at the same time? It goes back to our reliance on fake food, which typically has a lot of calories but very few vitamins, minerals and antioxidants—the essentials for building a healthy body. For example, a snack bag of Fritos Original Corn Chips contains 160 calories per ounce. If a kid eats a bag three times a week for a year, that adds up to 24,960 calories and potentially 8 pounds of weight gain. An apple containing only 65 calories and 3 grams of fiber is a much better snack option.

The formula for body weight is simple. More calories *in* (food) and fewer calories *out* (activity) lead to weight gain. The opposite is also true. Fewer calories taken in from food and more calories out from physical activity result in weight loss. So overconsumption of fake foods that are high in calories can quite easily increase a child's total daily caloric intake. Combine these excess calories with a sedentary lifestyle, and you end up with overweight or obese children who haven't eaten a single fruit or vegetable containing the essential nutrients their bodies need to grow and develop.

HEALTHY BODIES, HEALTHY MINDS

The absence of nutrient-rich foods in kids' diets has perpetuated strong preferences for fast food and processed foods, and an equal dislike of fruits and vegetables. This trend in youth eating habits has sparked the attention of a number of grassroots, government, and private organizations focused on improving the health of America. Healthy People 2010 is a set of health objectives designed to identify the most significant preventable health threats to our nation. The initiative is charged with establishing national goals that encompass specific steps individuals, communities, and professionals can take to reduce these health threats. Healthy People 2010 has two main goals: 1) Increase the quality and years of healthy life, and 2) eliminate health disparities. One way to accomplish these goals is to have at least 75 percent of Americans eating at least two fruits daily. Yet the Centers for Disease Control (CDC) reports that only 32 percent of children in grades 9 to 12 are meeting this goal, and not without consequence: Action for Healthy Kids—the nation's leading nonprofit and largest volunteer network dedicated to fighting childhood obesity and undernourishment by partnering with schools to improve nutrition and physical activity—reports that 16 percent (or 9 million) of school-aged children and adolescents are overweight.

According to the CDC, kids haven't always been this heavy; in fact, the number of overweight kids has tripled since 1980. As a result of the increase in childhood obesity, the CDC estimates that 1 in 3 children will develop diabetes in their lifetime. Statistics from the National Diabetes Information Clearinghouse estimates the national cost of diabetes in one recent year exceeded $174 billion. Of this amount, $116 billion was due to excess medical expenditures and $58 billion in reduced national productivity attributed to diabetes.

BELIEVE IT OR NOT
In the 1940s, military recruits were being turned down because they didn't weigh enough. Today, they are being turned away because they weigh too much.

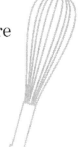

Not only is our health-care system feeling the effect of diabetes, but indirect costs resulting from increased absenteeism and reduced productivity are hitting our education system hard. Many studies have documented a strong link between healthy minds and healthy bodies. These studies point to a direct link between

childhood obesity facts

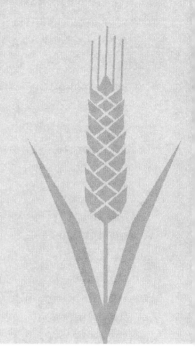

- 1 in 3 kids in this country are overweight or obese.
- Overweight and obese children, especially those in the teenage years, have a 70 percent chance of being obese as adults.
- Overweight and obese children with two obese parents have an 80 percent chance of becoming obese adults.
- Obesity causes many major health problems later in life.
- The rate of childhood obesity has more than doubled in children aged 2–5 and 12–19. The rate has more than tripled in kids aged 6–11.
- Poor diet and physical inactivity at school and at home are the major causes of childhood obesity.

Source: Centers for Disease Control and Robert Wood Johnson Foundation

nutritional intake and academic performance and between physical activity and academic achievement. Other research also suggests an association between weight problems and lower academic achievement. The negative effect on academic performance in overweight kids is includes increased absences resulting from physical, psychological or social problems brought on by poor nutrition, inactivity and weight problems. Bottom line: Healthy kids learn better because they are able to go to school, pay attention, and perform better in class.

IT STARTS WITH YOU

The days of not giving serious thought to the food our kids are eating is over. Becoming a mom inspired me to up the ante on good nutrition. Until my son was born, I had only my own nutritional needs to worry about. But having him changed everything. If you're a parent, I'm sure you feel the same need to provide only the best for your children. But the fact remains that modern family eating habits and inactivity have contributed to kids' inheriting poor eating habits and poor health. That's why we can no longer leave it up to television commercials or food manufacturers to guide us toward the best foods for our families. It's time to leave the "herd" I discussed in Chapter 3 and make some conscious choices about the food we eat and the example we're setting for our kids. Many kids haven't learned how to recognize and choose good food. They're relying on parents and other adult role models to set an example. Good nutrition and healthy living aren't discussed in many households, and public schools are forced to spend nearly all their instructional time on subject matter mandated by the No Child Left Behind Act. As a result, most kids don't learn the connection between their eating habits and their health.

Consider this snapshot into the eating habits of a group of teens I met recently. As a volunteer with the National 4-H Organization on the Healthy Lifestyles initiative, I had the opportunity last year to accompany a group of local teens to the first 4-H Force of 100 healthy living summit, a project funded by the Wal-Mart Foundation and sponsored by the National 4-H Council and local Cooperative Extension Centers. This project brought together almost 100 teenage students from across North Carolina to learn skills to be leaders in the fight to reduce obesity, stroke, heart disease, and diabetes in their communities.

BELIEVE IT OR NOT

The March 2010 issue of *Health Affairs* reported that children in the United States are heavy snackers, consuming candy, chips and other junk foods almost continuously throughout the day. These calories are consumed in addition to their regular meals.

The teens spent three days on the campus of North Carolina Agricultural and Technical State University learning how to read food labels, deciphering the fat and sugar content of their favorite fast-food meals, and understanding the role of unhealthy food in disease promotion. The teens and facilitators talked openly about the lifestyle risk factors for common diseases, such as diabetes, high blood pressure, and cancer, and their negative impact on sufferers' quality of life.

Right after lunch on the first day of the summit, the facilitator found herself trying to engage what looked like a group of teenage zombies. As I looked around the room, I could see that nearly half the kids had their heads down on their tables, while roughly another 25 percent were slumped back with their heads resting on the chair. The more the facilitator asked questions and shared moving stories as an effort to try and hold the teens' attention, the more they withdrew. They acted as if they had been drugged. During the break, I asked the facilitator if she would take a poll for me to determine what the kids had eaten during lunch. I was curious to know if they had eaten a lot of refined carbohydrates, such as pizza, chips, and ice cream, which cause a steep drop in blood sugar shortly after they are eaten. During the next hands-on activity, the facilitator asked the kids to line up across the room according to what they had eaten for lunch.

"Will everyone who ate pizza for lunch line up on the right side of the room?" the facilitator yelled. About half the kids got up and walked across the room. Then she asked for all the kids who had eaten fries, but no pizza, to line up along the front of the room. Another 30 percent of the students got up. Finally, anyone who had eaten a vegetable, but no pizza or fries, at lunch was asked to make their way to the left wall. Not surprisingly, the kids with their heads on their desks or slumped in their chairs were the exact ones who had eaten way too much processed food for lunch less than an hour earlier. When all was said and done, only about 15 percent of the kids were standing in the "vegetable, no-processed food group"; and, yes, nearly all these students were awake and alert during the afternoon presentations.

This simple, impromptu exercise evolved into an organic discussion about the connection between food and health, which helped the students recognize the mental and physical impact of food choices. They were able to correlate feeling sleepy and unfocused with the quality of food they ate for lunch. Their food choices had left many of them nonfunctional for more than an hour, and as a result, their learning potential was diminished during a highly informative presentation.

> "To keep the body in good health is a duty; otherwise
> we shall not be able to keep our mind strong and clear."
> **GAUTAMA THE BUDDHA**

At the end of our discussion about the kids' lunchtime food choices, they were polled again to see how many were willing to make a least one healthy change in their lunch options the following day. Only about 10 kids raised their hands. When the other 90 percent were asked what was preventing them from taking one small step toward a better outcome for the next day's class, the replies were astonishing: "This is what we always eat," "this is what we are used to eating at school and at home," *and* "this is what we like."

Most youth and teens I know love to eat pizza, hot dogs, burgers, fries, chicken nuggets, chips, and other highly processed foods. I wondered if what I was witnessing among the teens at this summit was a reflection of kids in classrooms after lunch all across America.

QUICK WINS TIPS

When you prepare and cook meals at home, you control the quality and quantity of the food your family eats.

Kids can't learn well if they don't have nutritious food to provide them with the energy and mental clarity to make it through the day. Once my son started elementary school, I became very concerned with the food he was getting during the school day in the form of cafeteria lunches, classroom snacks, and celebrations. The amount of processed food and sugar kids can potentially get at school is alarming. Parents, schools, and communities must work together to reform kids' meals and teach them skills that will make them more nutritionally aware of what they are eating. If we ever hope to reclaim the health and academic performance of our kids, we must expand the availability of nutritious food at home and at school.

JOIN THE CREW

As previously stated, this generation of children is predicted to be the first generation not expected to outlive their parents. But this is just a prediction—working together, parents, schools, communities, and the government can help change the course of children's health. During my son's first week of elementary school, I inquired about joining the school wellness council. A few days earlier he had brought home a cafeteria menu, which mentioned this council, describing it as a partnership between teachers, parents, school administrators, and the community to promote healthy eating and physical activity during the school day. It was the first week of school—and a brand-new school at that—and a School Wellness Council (SWC) hadn't been assembled. The school principal suggested I work with the Alliance for a Healthier Generation to start a volunteer council made up of individuals from the school and community who were dedicated to the development, implementation, and evaluation of school nutrition and physical activity practices and policies that promote a healthy school environment for students and staff. A joint venture between the American Heart Association and the Clinton Foundation, the Alliance for a Healthier Generation has a mission to eliminate childhood obesity by 2015.

In October 2008, our SWC was founded. Throughout the school year, with support from the Alliance's Healthy Schools Program North Carolina relationship manager, as well as other local resources, the SWC made great strides toward increasing access to nutritious foods in the cafeteria and in the classroom as well as providing more physical activity opportunities before and during school. Our school was moving at lightning speed—establishing a healthy snack and beverage list for parents, incorporating healthy living tips into the morning announcements and school newsletter, starting a before-school exercise program for students, planning for a school walking trail, and offering monthly nutrition promotions and contests. By the end of the school year, our school had met the requirements for the Healthy Schools Program bronze-level recognition. Our school principal and physical education teacher, both members of the SWC, were flown to New York to receive the award.

QUICK WINS TIPS

- Offer your children fruit, vegetables, nuts and whole grains instead of junk food.

- Ask your children's doctor to calculate their BMI percentile. If they're overweight or obese, take steps to ensure, in an encouraging and supportive manner, that they eat healthier and are physically active each day.

- Purge your kitchen and pantry of unhealthy snacks to cut the amount of fatty, salty and sugary foods in your children's diet.

To inspire other parents to become involved in wellness initiatives in their local schools, I was invited, along with another health-conscious mom from Nebraska, to join former President Bill Clinton on the *Rachael Ray Show* in May 2009 ("Walk the Walk" episode). After our appearance with Rachael Ray, we traveled to the Clinton Foundation offices to record a special Mother's Day Message with the president to promote healthy habits for children (http://tinyurl.com/okehd8). Meeting President Clinton was a once-in-a-lifetime experience—one I will never forget. I continue to be involved in activities at my son's school, North Carolina Action for Healthy Kids, North Carolina Parent Teacher Association, and other organizations to help create healthy home and school environments that promote nutritious eating and physical activity.

Our nation's First Mom, Michelle Obama, is also raising much-needed awareness about the rise and impact of childhood obesity through the Let's Move! Campaign (www.letsmove.gov). The Alliance for a Healthier Generation is a supporter of the Let's Move initiative. The goal of the campaign is simple yet colossal—to eradicate childhood obesity in one generation. Mrs. Obama has elevated the conversation about childhood obesity to franchise sports, chefs, parents, schools, and government. The initiative has accelerated action toward creating a society where health, wellness, prevention and disease management are paramount. Most notably, Mrs. Obama is setting a personal example of healthy living for children and parents across this country. We've all seen the First Mom planting and harvesting garden vegetables, playing Double Dutch, hula-hooping and eating fresh produce. These are things any parent can do.

The first lady is working to unite what I call an "Obesity Demolition Crew" to break down the barriers to healthy eating and active living that are threatening the livelihood of American children and their families. If you are a parent, work in a school, live in a community, or are an elected official, you're automatically a part of the Obesity Demolition Crew. What can you do as part of this demolition crew? Check out the "Obesity Demolition Crew Duties" chart on page 63 for a few ideas.

LEAD BY EXAMPLE

Kids want to be inspired. They want to live a long and healthy life. They need parents to change their relationship with food and demonstrate that real food—not processed, nutrient-poor alternatives—and optimal health are priorities. No parents want their children to inherit a lifestyle that promotes disease. So let's all do our part to ensure instead that all children in this country inherit an insatiable spirit for life, as well as the health to attain the life skills they need to be relevant in the 21st century and beyond. Our kids need us to choose a different path. There are many simple steps you can take to inspire and empower your kids to live healthier. Which step will you take today?

1. *Learn how to read and interpret food labels.* Then teach your kids.

2. *Set food rules.* Rules help children learn skills and behaviors to live successfully. Establish guidelines on the number of sweet treats to eat per day or per week and commit to serving at least one vegetable each night for dinner.

3. *Go Mediterranean.* The Mediterranean style of eating is deemed one of the healthiest in the world—rich in fresh fruits, vegetables, whole grains, fish, olive

OBESITY DEMOLITION CREW DUTIES

Parents

- Leave the "clean plate club"—allow children to stop eating when they are full rather than when their plate is empty. As kids get older, teach them to continue to rely on their inner wisdom to recognize when they're full.
- Cook more healthful meals at home at least three days a week. Use low-fat methods, such as baking, broiling, boiling, or microwaving, rather than frying.
- Set a good example by making smart food choices and being physically active.
- Provide kids with a healthy breakfast before each school day.
- Exercise with kids for at least 60 minutes on most days.
- Reduce sedentary, nonactive activities like watching television and play video games.
- Limit access to calorie-dense, nutrient-poor junk food (e.g., packaged snacks).
- Teach children how to recognize and resist savvy marketing strategies for unhealthy foods (e.g., sugar-laden kids' cereals).
- Become a volunteer in your child's school and in Action for Healthy Kids.
- Provide opportunities for kids to try new fruits and vegetables.
- Join your kids' School Wellness Council. If they don't have one, ask to start one!

Schools

- Offer a lot more natural, whole foods during breakfast and lunch and a lot fewer processed foods for all students.
- Support a School Wellness Council.
- Ensure all kids get at least 30 minutes of physical activity during each school day.
- Provide structured, active recess periods.
- Remove all vending machines from school property, unless they sell only healthy options like water, nuts, low-fat milk, and 100-percent-fruit juices.
- Encourage staff to be healthy role models for students.
- Promote and support parent involvement.
- Find creative ways to teach that incorporate nutrition and active living lessons.
- Enforce healthy school snacks.
- Start and provide ongoing support for a community garden.

Community

- Eliminate food desserts and increase access to healthy food for all citizens.
- Limit the growth of fast food restaurants in low-income communities.
- Increase walking-trail access to local schools.
- Increase public school funding.
- Increase funding and community access to parks and walking trails.

Government

- Continuously support increased funding for the Child Nutrition and WIC Reauthorization Act.
- Support funding for increased physical activity programs in schools.

oil, nuts, and moderate amounts of low-fat dairy. Kids love pizza, right? Fortunately, pizza is a great Mediterranean crossover food to incorporate into your family's meal plan. Instead of the traditional "put-you-to-sleep" pizza, introduce your kids to whole-wheat crusts topped with a variety of natural toppings, such as olives, fresh tomatoes, onions, mushrooms, peppers, basil, garlic, and other fresh ingredients. Check out *The Mediterranean Diet Cookbook* (Bantam) by Nancy Harmon Jenkins for a history of the Mediterranean culture and cuisine as well as a variety of great, simple recipes.

4. *Eat more home-cooked meals.* Cooking meals at home is the best way to save money and control portion sizes, quality of ingredients, and salt and trans-fat content. Home-cooked meals also provide an excellent opportunity for families to eat together and establish a tradition of home cooking. In addition to improving eating habits, studies show that eating meals together increases communication and improves kids' academic performance.

5. *Expand your knowledge of healthier food choices.* It's not too late to start making better food and lifestyle choices, and it's definitely not too late to make a difference in your kids' lives. Read and research to learn all you can about better ways to eat and solutions to common challenges for families. Then share what you know to inspire other families to eat more whole, organically grown plant foods, and less chemically processed animal and junk foods.

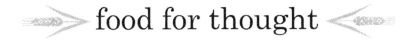

food for thought

- Don't let food manufacturers and marketing campaigns dictate what you feed your family. Use your wisdom to guide you toward real food.

- A lithium test for real food: Ask yourself if your great-grandmother would recognize it as food and eat it herself.

- Get involved in your home, in your child's school, and in community organizations to promote healthy eating and physical activity as a normal way of life.

- Being a parent means sometimes you'll have to say "no" to foods that aren't good for your kids, even if "all" their friends can have it.

TRADING IN YOUR OLD LIFESTYLE

So you're thinking about trading in your old eating habits for a newer, healthier set of behaviors. You've carefully considered all the reasons it's time to get rid of your old eating habits. They're draining your energy, making your clothes fit uncomfortably, causing you to miss time from work due to illness, and wreaking havoc on your finances. You've done your research: After spending a great deal of time reading information in magazines, blogs, books, online forums, and websites about the new behaviors you're considering, you ask a few friends who already

> "Limitations live only in our minds. But if we use our imaginations, our possibilities become limitless."
> **JAMIE PAOLINETTI**

have the habits you want about their experiences. They all have only great things to say about the behaviors you're thinking about adopting.

You now have all the information you need to support your decision to purge your old habits. Although you know it will be hard to get rid of these habits because they've been with you since you were a kid—in fact, your parents gave them to you—without further delay, you take the plunge. You embark upon a healthier life full of abundant energy, optimal health, and exciting, flavorful natural foods —and you don't look back.

SNAP OUT OF IT!

Changing the habits you've had all your life can be scary. The unfamiliarity of the unknown can be enough to deter you from doing what you know is in your best interest. You envision the change being too hard to make, because the transition will take you out of your comfort zone. You'll have to change your routine. You may have to do things you've never done before. You may have to engage in activities you don't like very much in order to attain the goals you've set for yourself. Just the thought of making these changes frightens you.

To cross the imaginary finish line we alluded to in Chapter 1, you'll have to press on through the fear of change. But the fear makes you feel stuck. Have you ever heard the saying, "the only way out is through"? This means the only way you can get past the uneasy feelings you have about transforming your life is to get focused, get determined and get through it. Realizing you can still move forward, despite being fearful and unsure, is hugely motivating. You know there's nothing standing in your way. Armed with this motivation, you're equipped to move mountains! Speaking of mountains, let's discuss the biggest mountain you may potentially face as you begin changing your lifestyle and the negative effect it can have on you.

POWER OF THE POSITIVE

Do you believe that certain tasks are impossible for you to achieve, that you don't have what it takes to succeed, or that you're destined for failure? Do you ever say to yourself, "I can never do that"? Most of us have probably encountered these thoughts at some point in our lives. This behavior is the result of self-limiting beliefs or mindsets. Self-limiting beliefs are mental blocks or negative self-talk that limits your ability to achieve your goals. These negative thoughts are harmful to you because they can cause you to dismiss or talk yourself out of realistic and attainable goals.

QUICK WINS TIPS

Recognizing the self-limiting beliefs that take up residence in your mind creates an opportunity for you to minimize their effect on your life. Once you identify self-limiting beliefs, immediately take action to:

° Turn procrastination into proactive action.

° Turn dampened spirits into moments of hope.

° Turn distractions from your goals into determination to meet your goals.

The most important quality you must possess to be successful in achieving anything you desire is the capacity to believe in yourself. You must be your biggest cheerleader and a staunch advocate for your capabilities and potential. Self-limiting beliefs are destructive, because they tear down this fundamental level of self-development. So how can you protect yourself against these inner gremlins?

If you want to be successful in life, you can't afford to entertain negative thoughts for even a second. Your greatest weapon against self-limiting beliefs is awareness. By recognizing the self-doubt as soon as it creeps into your consciousness, you have the power to dismiss it immediately. You can easily clear the negativity out of your head by replacing the thought with a positive affirmation, or a statement to manifest change. Positive affirmations are most effective at triggering positive action when they're repeated many times. Positive affirmations have helped countless people develop positive self-talk and a can-do attitude. Here are several common self-limiting beliefs you should be aware of:

SELF-LIMITING BELIEF	» POSITIVE AFFIRMATION
I am not good enough.	» Everything I need is already within me.
This is impossible for me to achieve.	» I can do anything I set my mind to do.
I am destined to fail.	» I am successful in whatever I do.
I am not capable of success.	» I deserve to be happy, healthy, and successful.
I can't achieve anything great.	» I prosper wherever I turn.

Author and poet David Herbert Lawrence illustrated the magnificent power of the mind with this quote: "The mind can assert anything and pretend it has proved it." The bright side of this coin is that thoughts can work two ways—to build you up or tear you down. Choose to tap into your phenomenal mental power to plan, act, and achieve your healthy-eating goals. Remember, you can achieve anything you set your mind to. A healthier lifestyle is built one healthy habit at a time.

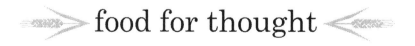

food for thought

○ Limitations on what you can achieve begin and end in your mind.

○ To change or not to change. That is the question.

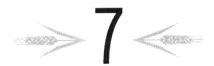

FROM DREAMS TO RESULTS

Perhaps when I mentioned the notion of herd behavior in Chapter 3, you wondered if there are situations where following a herd can actually work in your favor. The answer is yes. It wasn't until I started hanging out with someone more health conscious than I that I started to reconsider my own lifestyle behaviors.

It is never too late to re-evaluate your lifestyle and make the choice to do things a bit differently. In this chapter, you'll discover how to move past obstacles and gain the momentum you need to achieve the health goals you've set for yourself and your family. You'll see how the power of relying on the strength and knowledge of others, tapping into your creativity, and connecting with your greatest motivators can turn your dreams into a reality.

TWO ARE BETTER THAN ONE

My husband, Michael, continued to exercise regularly after he left the military. His fitness routine varied. Some days he would hit the gym after work. Other days he would get up early before work to jog a few miles. It was hard for me to stay in bed after he had gotten up early to jog or lift weights, because lying there made me feel like such a slacker. But more so, I really enjoyed doing things with my husband, and exercising with him was no exception.

Fortunately for me, my significant other was a motivator. But what if your spouse or other family member is a couch potato? Where will you seek support for the changes you and your family need to make? You have some choices to make. I recommend you find someone else to be your motivator if you can't motivate your family to join you. Before you help others, you have to help yourself. Once you begin to change the way you eat and exercise regularly, your family will notice. Do you have a friend, co-worker or neighbor who's conscientious about her diet and exercises regularly? If so, ask if she would be willing to be your workout buddy, or at the very least, an accountability partner to help you stay on track with your own goals. If she's health-conscious, I'd bet she'd be willing to help you develop healthier habits. Perhaps she has some tips to share on ways she gets her kids to try new foods. You could even swap healthy recipes. An accountability partner doesn't even have to live near you. A friend of mine has an accountability partner who calls her every morning at 5:15 am to make sure she's up and ready to workout with an exercise video before she heads out herself to a nearby gym. They also exchange recipes and healthy snack ideas via email.

Every time I followed Michael to the gym, I benefited. I became more and more comfortable in the gym environment. Soon, I gained enough confidence to take spinning and step-aerobics classes.

BELIEVE IT OR NOT

You're more likely to stick with an exercise program or healthy-eating goals when friends or family members participate with you.

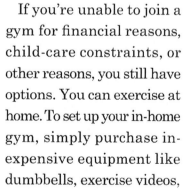

If you're unable to join a gym for financial reasons, child-care constraints, or other reasons, you still have options. You can exercise at home. To set up your in-home gym, simply purchase inexpensive equipment like dumbbells, exercise videos, yoga mats, and resistance bands from Wal-Mart or Target. You could also see if there's a used sports equipment store nearby, like Play It Again Sports, which offers reasonably priced treadmills, elliptical machines, and stationary bikes. And nothing beats a brisk walk outdoors if you live in a safe neighborhood with good sidewalks. Another friend of mine gets really creative with fitting in exercise on days when she can't squeeze in a "formal" workout by marching in place while she washes dishes or folds laundry. Where there's a will, there's a way!

IF IT WAS TO BE, IT WAS UP TO ME

When I started exercising at the gym with my husband, my first stop was the treadmill. To me, it seemed like the easiest machine to tackle. And when I felt comfortable enough, I started jogging. At first, I absolutely hated jogging. Self-limiting beliefs started creeping into my mind, telling me I couldn't do it. With every pounding step, I thought back to when I gave up on athletics back in high school. That's when I quit the cheerleading squad because I was too embarrassed of my fat, jiggly thighs. If I had continued to pursue sports back then, I reasoned, my body wouldn't be suffering from such physical shock in my late 20s. Although I was a bit embarrassed to be huffing and puffing so hard on the treadmill and lagging so far behind others in aerobics class, I refused to listen to the negative thoughts telling me to quit.

> "Act as if what you do makes a difference. It does."
> **WILLIAM JAMES**

In a recent *Essence* magazine interview, President Obama and the first lady shared their views on their daughters' education. The couple expressed that earning a "B" isn't good enough in their household, because there's no reason why their daughters can't earn "A's." I didn't give up on changing my eating habits, because I knew there was no reason I couldn't succeed. If it was to be, it was up to me. (By the way, this is a great affirmation.) I wouldn't give up because I wanted to avoid the obesity-related health problems that affect many of my family members. My mother, father, auntie, and paternal grandmother have high blood pressure. Another auntie has diabetes. My maternal grandmother and four of her siblings died from various forms of cancer. Having studied biology extensively in college and graduate school, I was well aware of how the body worked. I knew if I wanted to ward off the obesity-related diseases hanging on my family tree, I would have to eat smarter and exercise regularly. So each day I tried to jog just a few steps farther than I had the time before. And when I got tired of jogging (and that certainly didn't take long), I walked the remaining minutes of my treadmill program.

When I first began this journey toward changing a lifetime of habits, I had to intentionally stay in a mental space that celebrated my extra energy, increased flexibility, and empowerment. Otherwise my thoughts would have been consumed with all the changes I had to make to live healthier, and I would have certainly grown frustrated and eventually given up. Unfortunately, in our society the unhealthy choice is the cheapest and most convenient one. I knew if good food and good health was to be a reality in my life, it was up to me. I often used positive affirmations as discussed in Chapter 6 to keep me encouraged.

One of my favorite affirmations, "I can do all things through Christ, who strengthens me," comes from the Bible. Affirmations were—and still—remain valuable Quick Wins for me. Maybe they can serve as support for you, too.

QUICK WINS TIPS

Here are some affirmations I use that shift negative thoughts into positive realities:

- I choose to enjoy this moment.

- I am positive and confident.

- I choose to be healthy and happy.

- Each day I am in control of my food choices.

- My life is important.

- I love life.

REPLACEMENT THERAPY

It's possible to make great strides toward changing a habit once you stop negative self-talk. When we feel a little pull against our will, we tell ourselves things like "skipping one day of exercise won't matter" or "I'll eat this piece of chocolate cake because I deserve it." Or here's a good one: "I'll burn off these cookies later on the treadmill." Is this pattern of rationalizing familiar to you? If you repeatedly give in to these types of thoughts, they can quickly derail your attempts at living a healthy and happy life. Before you know it, you will have reverted back to your old habits, because they're more familiar and therefore easier to maintain.

Replacing negative, self-defeating thoughts about healthier eating with new, positive information is a proven way to support an improved lifestyle. So devour all the information you can get your hands on from books, cooking and fitness magazines, websites, cookbooks, workshops, and cooking demonstrations that offer practical ways—in addition to those offered in this book—to help you fit good food into your lifestyle.

To be successful, you'll need to transition from highly processed foods to fruits, veggies, nuts, yogurt and other

BELIEVE IT OR NOT
The White House wants your family to be healthy, too! The President's Council on Fitness, Sports & Nutrition recommends being active with family and friends as one of its "Top 10 Tips for Healthy Eating and Physical Activity." Visit www.fitness.gov/10tips.htm for the other nine tips.

nourishing alternatives. This transition will require you to prepare more meals at home. I know cooking at home has become nonexistent in many American families, but it's a basic foundational principle that needs to find its way back into American culture. Learning to cook and prepare your meals and snacks will have the most significant positive impact on your eating habits. When you prepare your own meals, you have more control over the ingredients and their quality.

On average, I cook about four days per week, and on most other days we eat leftovers. We either order take-out or dine out about once a week, usually on the weekends. My family is used to it. They know that 90 percent of the time Mom is going to opt for eating something from home.

Cooking is doable when you establish a system that supports meal preparation. If you're a novice or short on time, chose recipes with a handful of familiar ingredients and few preparation steps. Generally, the simpler the recipe and ingredients, the better it is for you in terms of convenience and nutrition. Simplicity is an indication that the ingredients are close to their natural form.

As I stated in Chapter 2, my food philosophy is that food should taste good, nourish the body, and preserve health. That's why today I opt for dishes that are simple, natural, and delicious. My favorite cuisine is Mediterranean. I love how traditional Mediterranean fare is rich in succulent olive oil, fresh fruits and vegetables, and nuts, and scarce in amounts of meat. You can learn more about the benefits of the Mediterranean way of eating in Chapter 8.

But for now, let's get back to my Southern eating roots. I was raised by a family of traditional cooks who were highly skilled at making food taste good. I grew up on the best fried chicken, seasoned collards, potatoes, cornbread, and rich pound cakes. So naturally I was at a huge loss when I began trying to learn healthier ways to prepare meals. When I got stuck in the middle of a recipe calling for fresh herbs or a cooking technique I was unfamiliar with, who could I call? And then there was my apprehension about whether this "new" food would taste as good as the foods I was familiar with. This is a time when those positive affirmations came in handy to help me stick to my mission. I would say to myself, "I enjoy healthy, delicious, and balanced meals." One day while cooking, I overheard Joyce Meyer on an *Enjoying Everyday Life* broadcast say that in order for us to succeed in life, we must "learn to walk through our fear." At that moment, I knew if I wanted to live happier and healthier, I had to walk, jog, weight train, and cook nutritious meals amidst the fear.

As I continued to walk through my fear of leaving old, familiar, and comfortable habits behind while embracing new, healthier, and sometimes challenging habits, I began to notice a connection between my food and my health. When I ate wholesome, natural food like fruits, vegetables, whole grains, and lean protein, I seemed to have more energy to help me get through the day. However, when I overindulged on refined sugars like chocolate brownies, candy bars, and white bread, I felt bloated, tired, and cranky. As I developed a greater understanding of the way the food I eat impacts the mind and body, I began to see a much bigger paradigm taking shape. Healthy eating changed my life and empowered me to overcome fear and take hold of little bits of progress that led me each day toward a healthier, more secure future.

Take notice of how you feel immediately after eating certain foods. How is your energy, clarity of thoughts, mood, attention span, and learning potential immediately after you eat? If you can give each of these areas a "thumbs-up," then keep on eating what you're eating. But if you don't rank so well in these areas after eating, then a change in diet is in order. You should feel alive and exhilarated after eating—if you don't, you're eating the wrong foods. And if you're eating the wrong foods, your kids are most likely eating the wrong foods, too.

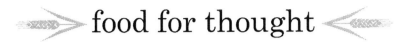

food for thought

- Get buy-in from family on the healthy changes they wish to make. Then hold each of them accountable, even the young ones, for making the changes they express an interest in making.

- Find an affirmation that resonates with you, or take a few moments to create your own. The words can serve as a great source of inspiration when you want to quit your healthy eating goals.

- Start a log to chronicle your journey, especially the good things you experience along the way, like a change in your energy level or a new food your child was willing to try. Use our Quick Wins Log in Appendix C, or create your own!

FOOD EMPOWERMENT

Empowerment is defined in Ken Blanchard's book *Leading at a Higher Level* as the process of unleashing the power in people—their knowledge, experience and motivation—and focusing that power to achieve positive outcomes. In his book, Blanchard provides guidance on leading people to greatness in the context of creating high-performing organizations. In this chapter, I will show you how to apply these basic concepts to liberate your authority and power to make empowered food choices. These choices will help you get more out of life—more health, more energy, and more freedom.

STAY IN CONTROL

Food empowerment, like so many things in life, involves both choice and control. Who's in charge of what you eat, anyway? You are, of course. But when we're bombarded by television and magazine ads and fast-paced lifestyles, it's so easy to give up our power in exchange for other preferences, like taste and convenience. Nonetheless, the question still stands: Is it worth sacrificing your health?

> "People already have power through their knowledge and motivation. The key to empowerment is letting this power out."
> **KEN BLANCHARD**

Food choices based exclusively on a single preference, like taste, are the hallmark of impulsive decision making. When taste dictates choice, our connections with food become limited and our opportunity to prevent disease is diminished. Conversely, when we take control of our impulse to overindulge in foods that taste good but are not necessarily good for us, we begin the transition toward a more redefined thought process. This process of conscious thinking is shaped by our knowledge, experience, and convictions, and it contributes to self-empowerment.

Webster defines "empowerment" as *the act of giving power or official authority to.* Self-empowerment is exhibited through our own authority and control to exercise behaviors that enable us to shape and reclaim our health. When we make food choices based on knowledge, experience, and conviction, we expand our realm of possibilities. When we base our food choices on taste alone, our possibilities are narrowed.

As you begin to tap into an empowering relationship with food, healthier choices will feel natural and appropriate because they're coming from more conscious thought. For instance, instead of afternoon, spur-of-the-moment craving trips to the vending machine for chips and a soda, you'll think about what you can eat that will support what you would really like to have, such as improved health, more energy, and greater longevity.

You may also begin to be more in tune with your body. For instance, you may start to notice how long you typically feel energized after a carbohydrate- and calorie-dense snack, like a candy bar, before your next energy slump hits. For most people, the slump occurs about an hour later. Once you realize that chips and soda are an easy, short-term fix for low energy, you'll be empowered to take steps to make your food work for you instead of against you.

The first step is to improve the quality of your meals and snacks throughout the day by incorporating more fruits, vegetables, whole grains, and lean protein. The second step is to spread out what you eat throughout the day to keep your energy levels steady. Impactful change doesn't require monumental shifts in behavior. Remember, Quick Wins lead to big changes. By making these empowered steps to change what, when, and how you eat, you can sustain your energy, feel better, and be more productive now and as you continue to age.

THE MAJOR CULPRITS

Obesity is a direct outcome of our propensity for consuming foods with too much salt, sugar, and fat. These culprits abound in our diets through processed and restaurant foods. Fat adds flavor, but it's the salty and sugary tastes that we're addicted to—and what we need to limit in our diets.

Salty, but Definitely not Sweet

When we want to eat, we instinctively want something that tastes good and is easy to get. Salt (sodium), a dietary mineral essential to human life, makes food

BEFORE YOU PUT IT ON YOUR PLATE, EVALUATE

Empowered food choices aren't based on a single factor, like taste, but are decisions resulting from a number of factors. Here are some questions—and answers—to help you evaluate your food choices.

Q: How will the calories in this meal impact my overall daily caloric intake?

A: Eating in moderation is key to sustaining a healthy-eating lifestyle. To make room in your diet for a splurge, ascertain the calories in the food you're eating by reading the nutrition label or checking the restaurant nutritional information. Factor these calories into the number of calories you need for the whole day, then determine how much you should eat.

Q: Is this food heavily processed (highly refined)?

A: In general, highly processed or unnatural foods contain a long list of ingredients that include the words "enriched" or "bleached," contain hard-to-pronounce words, spout bold marketing claims and were not available 200 years ago.

Q: Does this food contain preservatives or artificial additives?

A: The nutrition label includes a list of added preservatives or additives. Some common food additives you may see listed include sodium nitrate, cellulose, mannitol, Blue No. 1, Red No. 2, Red No. 40, Yellow No. 5, and guar gum. Visit the website for the Center for Science in the Public Interest (*www.cspinet.org/index.html*) for an extensive listing of common food additives.

Q: Is this food rich in antioxidants?

A: Natural, whole foods are a great source of beneficial antioxidants, natural food substances that rid the body of free radicals that can cause cellular damage and may contribute to chronic disease. Richly colored fruits and vegetables are rich in antioxidants. To get a healthy range of antioxidants, eat a variety of plant foods representing a rainbow of colors. Foods with high amounts of antioxidants include berries, spinach, tomatoes and red grapes.

taste really good. The taste of salt is so appealing and ubiquitous that most of us consume far more than we need. Most of this salt comes from ever-present junk foods, like chips, french fries, processed meats, and fast food. In fact, according to the American Heart Association and the Mayo Clinic, about 75 percent of sodium in the

American diet comes from hidden sources of sodium in packaged, processed restaurant food. While you're on the lookout for sodium in your diet, don't forget the salt you add to your food from salt shakers. Just look around the next time you're eating in a crowded restaurant to see how many people reach for the salt shaker before they reach for their fork.

Generally, the more processed a food item is, the more salt it contains. People who eat diets high in sodium typically have higher blood pressure, a major risk factor for heart disease and stroke. On the other hand, people who adopt ways to reduce their sodium consumption may benefit from improved blood pressure and reduce their risk of developing other serious chronic diseases.

To illustrate how easy it is to exceed the daily recommended allowance for salt, let's take a peek at the nutrition label for a "Grab Bag" of Lay's Original potato chips, which you've undoubtedly seen in convenience stores. While this 2-ounce bag of mostly air may seem like a sparse snack, it contains 330mg of sodium. Pair those chips with a turkey and ham sandwich, and you can find yourself quickly approaching

BELIEVE IT OR NOT
The average American eats roughly a gallon and an half of salt each year. This is equivalent to 1,152 teaspoons of salt! According to the Centers for Disease Control and Prevention, the average *daily* U.S. intake of sodium is 3,500mg, or 1½ teaspoons, with 77 percent of added sodium coming from processed foods.

the daily recommended allowance for sodium in one sitting. Go online (www.dietaryguidelines.gov) to access the current dietary guidelines and determine your recommended daily allowance of sodium as well as macronutrients—those required by the body in greater quantities—like carbohydrates, fats, and proteins appropriate for your age and health profile.

Remember, if you're eating something out of a box, can, or bag, you can easily determine how much salt it contains by looking at the nutrition label on the package. The nutrition label provides important information about food, such as serving size, servings per container, calories, and amounts of macronutrients, vitamins, and minerals.

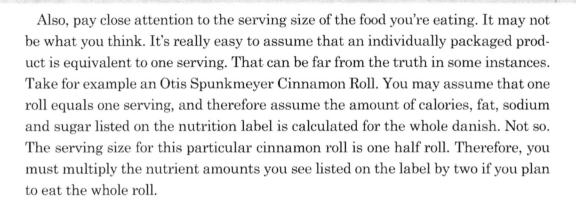

how much is enough?

According to the latest dietary guidelines for Americans, adults should consume less than 2,300mg (approximately 1 teaspoon of salt) of sodium per day. For people with chronic diseases like high blood pressure, diabetes, or kidney disease, as well as older adults and African Americans, the recommended daily limit is 1,500mg, or roughly half a teaspoon of salt.

Also, pay close attention to the serving size of the food you're eating. It may not be what you think. It's really easy to assume that an individually packaged product is equivalent to one serving. That can be far from the truth in some instances. Take for example an Otis Spunkmeyer Cinnamon Roll. You may assume that one roll equals one serving, and therefore assume the amount of calories, fat, sodium and sugar listed on the nutrition label is calculated for the whole danish. Not so. The serving size for this particular cinnamon roll is one half roll. Therefore, you must multiply the nutrient amounts you see listed on the label by two if you plan to eat the whole roll.

At first glance, you may not see any need for caution before ordering a McDonald's Premium Grilled Chicken Classic Sandwich, but you'll want to look at the nutrition label, especially if you're on a low-salt diet. According to McDonald's nutrition facts, which can be downloaded from its website, one grilled chicken sandwich contains 1,190mg of sodium, or 50 percent of the recommended daily value of sodium. By choosing this sandwich, in one meal you'll consume nearly half the salt needed for a whole day. Not only that, but if you answer "yes" when the cashier asks if you want an Extra Value Meal, then add another 350mg of sodium for the medium french fries you're about to eat. Wash your meal down with a medium Sprite, and you'll add another 55mg of sodium. This brings the sodium content to a grand total of approximately 1,595mg for a single meal—well over half the daily recommended allowance of 2,400mg suggested for the average American. And this doesn't even take into account other sodium-containing foods you're likely to eat throughout the day.

The Food and Drug Administration recognizes the impact of processed and packaged foods on the salt intake of Americans and plans to initiate the first legal limits on the amount of salt allowed in processed foods. The initiative is expected to be launched by the end of 2010. Officials have not yet determined the salt limits, but plans are underway to gradually reduce sodium intake from foods over the next several years.

KEYS TO SUCCESS

As you can tell, the key to managing your salt intake is reading food labels. Reading labels may seem intimidating and time consuming at first, but once you begin to understand the power of the information, you'll no longer want to eat food without knowing what's in it. It's prudent to evaluate nutrition facts for yourself rather than rely on food marketers for this information.

These examples of sodium-rich foods aren't provided to suggest that you avoid these foods altogether. Instead, they're highlighted to encourage you to become more conscious of your innate impulse for salt and to inspire you to make food choices that won't jeopardize your health.

BY ANY OTHER NAME

Note that added salt comes in many forms and may be listed on nutrition labels as monosodium glutamate (MSG), sodium nitrate, sodium nitrite, sodium saccharin, baking soda (sodium bicarbonate), and sodium benzoate.

Empowered food choices are healthier food choices. Eating foods close to their original source is the best way to control your salt intake and maintain a normal blood pressure. For example, choosing fresh fruits and vegetables like apples and carrots in their natural form to eat along with a sandwich is a better option than a side of highly processed foods like chips. Even though there will be times when fresh isn't possible, you can still make smart choices to give your body the vitamins, minerals, and antioxidants it needs without compromising your health. Begin preparing foods without added salt and ordering restaurant meals without any added salt.

Think about other ways you can reduce sodium in your daily diet. One approach could be a switch to more fiber-rich alternatives, such as fresh fruit, in situations where you usually eat salty chips. You might also brown-bag a healthfully prepared lunch a couple of days a week to cut back on high-sodium restaurant and fast food. Seek foods close to their source, prepare and cook meals at home as

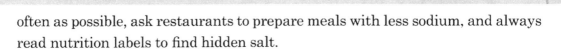

how much is enough?

Sodium chloride, or table salt, is approximately 40 percent sodium. Understand just how much sodium is in salt so you can take measures to control your intake.

1/4 teaspoon salt = 600mg sodium   1/2 teaspoon salt = 1,200mg sodium
3/4 teaspoon salt = 1,800mg sodium   1 teaspoon salt = 2,300mg sodium

Source: American Heart Association

often as possible, ask restaurants to prepare meals with less sodium, and always read nutrition labels to find hidden salt.

I'll bet you're wondering what you can eat for breakfast or lunch that's tasty but not loaded with salt. Many American favorites like breakfast biscuit sandwiches, bacon, and cheese won't fit the bill. A word of caution: Don't try to overhaul your diet all at once. Trying to tackle too many changes at one time may overwhelm you and increase the likelihood that you'll give up altogether and revert back to your old way of eating. Start with one or two Quick Wins. Once you master those, add a few more. Be practical and plan for your success.

Hey, Sugar

America's love affair with sugar is just as strong as its attraction to salt. As our love for sugar grows, so do our waistlines. As is the case with salt, our impulsive tendency to make food decisions based primarily on taste also results in our over-consumption of sugar.

It's probably no surprise that sugary drinks are the number-one source of excessive sugar in both adults and teenagers. To get a better picture of just how much sugar we really get from soft drinks, let's look at the nutrition facts for Amer-

BY ANY OTHER NAME

Did you catch the term "added sugar"? Added sugar isn't just the sugar you dip a spoon into to sweeten your coffee or cereal. The catch-all term "added sugar" also includes sweeteners and syrups added to food during processing and preparation to make them tastier. Added sugars may be listed as cane sugar, beet sugar, sucrose, corn syrup, high-fructose corn syrup, corn sugar, glucose, and honey. Added sugar is also found in some unexpected places, like crackers and bread.

ica's favorite soda, Coke, which, according to *Beverage Digest*, topped the 2009 Top-10 list of soft drink brands. According to the nutrition label for Coke, a typical 20-ounce bottle is about two servings. The serving size should serve as your first eye-opener. Did you have any idea that one bottle contained more than a single serving? That *one* serving contains 27 grams of sugar, or a little more than 6 teaspoons! Truth is, most Americans don't stop at just one serving but drink the whole bottle of cola, containing roughly 54 grams (13.5 teaspoons) of sugar. If you're a woman and you drink one 20-ounce bottle of Coke, you've already consumed more than two times the recommended daily allowance for sugar; and if you're a man, you've exceeded the daily allowance.

We're taught as young children to finish whatever our parents give us to eat or drink. As a result, our brains are ingrained with the belief that we're "done" when we've finished everything. This explains why it feels completely natural to stop drinking a Coke when the bottle is empty, whether it's a 12-ounce can or a 20-ounce bottle. Fortunately, it's easy to reset the brain's "done" signal by simply altering environmental cues like glass size. If you choose to have an occasional soda, take control of the amount you consume by drinking out of an 8-ounce glass, and don't go back for seconds!

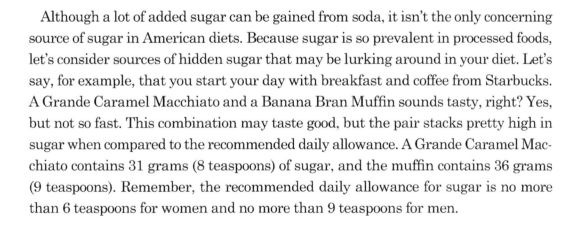

BELIEVE IT OR NOT
According to the American Heart Association, Americans gobble up an average of 22 teaspoons (1 teaspoon = 4 grams) of added sugar every day.

Although a lot of added sugar can be gained from soda, it isn't the only concerning source of sugar in American diets. Because sugar is so prevalent in processed foods, let's consider sources of hidden sugar that may be lurking around in your diet. Let's say, for example, that you start your day with breakfast and coffee from Starbucks. A Grande Caramel Macchiato and a Banana Bran Muffin sounds tasty, right? Yes, but not so fast. This combination may taste good, but the pair stacks pretty high in sugar when compared to the recommended daily allowance. A Grande Caramel Macchiato contains 31 grams (8 teaspoons) of sugar, and the muffin contains 36 grams (9 teaspoons). Remember, the recommended daily allowance for sugar is no more than 6 teaspoons for women and no more than 9 teaspoons for men.

KEYS TO SUCCESS

Remember from our earlier discussion that the more processed a food is, the more salt it contains? Well, the same rule applies to sugar. Processed foods rich in sugar and saturated fats, like cookies and cakes, are *calorie dense* and provide little to no nutritive value. *Nutrient-dense* foods like low-fat milk, fresh fruit and

how much is enough?

The American Heart Association recommends that women who eat a balanced diet consisting of about 2,000 calories per day consume less than 6 teaspoons (24 grams or 100 calories) of added sugar per day. Men are allowed a little more sugar than women, roughly 9 teaspoons (36 grams or 150 calories) of added sugar per day. You see, there is room for sugar in a healthful diet. However, too much added sugar is a threat to optimal health.

some vegetables also contain sugar, but these natural sugars offer the body beneficial nutrients, unlike added sugars that simply provide empty calories. Practice seeking out foods with natural sugars like fructose and lactose (fruit sugar and milk sugar) that provide nourishment to the body. Appendix D provides a brief list of nutrient- and calorie-dense foods to help you recognize and integrate more sugar-conscious foods into your diet.

You can also find information at a great website called SugarStacks.com, which provides striking visuals of just how much sugar is found in some common foods and beverages. Visit the site to find out where sugar is hiding in some of your favorite breads, breakfast cereals and salad dressings. Books like *The South Beach Diet, You on a Diet,* and websites with accurate, credible information, like WebMD, are other great resources. You can find more information on the internet. Good keywords to use in a Google search include "sugar dietary guidelines," "low-glycemic index foods," and "sugar-conscious recipes."

CREATING A LIFESTYLE

Healthy eating is more important than most people realize. The foods we eat regularly can strengthen our health, or they can take away from it, leading to diseases like The Big Four (as discussed in Chapter 4). People unwilling to change their eating habits will argue that genetics plays a big role in whether diseases manifest in the body. Genes do play a role in disease formation, but studies show that lifestyle plays an even greater role in chronic disease than genetics, as much as 70 percent. You're creating your lifestyle with every bite of food.

I don't mean to trivialize our attraction to salty and sweet tastes. It's important for the food we eat to be tasty; otherwise we won't want it. Many years ago, when humans foraged the earth for food, unpleasant tastes often protected them from ingesting deadly berries and leaves and led them to the nutrients their bodies needed. Ironically, the taste impulses that once protected us are now leading us to danger through excessive food consumption. Fortunately, our ability for conscious thought is our saving grace. It's when modern impulses for unhealthy foraging attempt to overpower us that we must tap into our evolved power of conscious thought to recognize and circumvent cravings that aren't in the best interest of our well-being.

Individuals who feel empowered (i.e., believe they have the authority and control to improve their lives) are driven to look a little deeper, ask a few more questions, and take different paths to do what's best for optimal health. They believe small dietary changes are possible in their own lives, and they make strides toward improving their health.

to tell the truth

When searching the web for accurate, credible health-related information, keep the following six tips in mind during your evaluation:

1. Does the website address start with http:// and end in .gov, .us, .edu, .org, or .(abbreviation for the state)?

2. Does it clearly state who's responsible for the site and its information (e.g., USDA)?

3. Have the web pages been updated recently? The "published" or "updated" date can usually be found at the bottom of the page.

4. Is the information based on factual data, rather than the author's opinion? If the article is written in first person and includes sentences such as "I think" or "In my opinion," those are red flags. Statements that cite experts or research are more credible.

5. Does the site provide a clear statement of purpose? This will help you ascertain the intention of the site's owner.

6. Can you find the contact information and additional resources for more information?

In my experience, embracing healthy change was easier once I discovered my personal connection to eating more nutritious foods. My motive became more than just the desire to lose weight. Many people learn the hard way that weight, in and of itself, is not a compelling reason to change lifestyle habits and soon revert back to old habits. I really connect with the nutritional aspects of food. I believe in the power of simple, nutritious food that's close to its original source (natural food) to nourish the body and promote health. I want to live a happy, healthy, vibrant, and long life, and I believe wholeheartedly that paying closer attention to the food I put into my body will help me attain the vision I have for my life.

I want to inspire others to do the same. My vision is that others will make the connection between food and health and feel confident enough to live by that philosophy throughout their everyday lives.

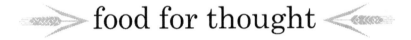

food for thought

○ The more processed a food is, the more salt and sugar it contains.

○ It's easier to manage the quality of your food when you prepare it yourself.

○ It's too easy to exceed the daily recommended limits for salt, sugar and fat if you eat the Standard American Diet.

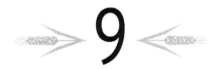

CREATING AND EXECUTING A FOOD PHILOSOPHY

When I work with wellness-coaching clients who are striving to reclaim their health and overall sense of well-being, they often begin the journey by creating a food philosophy or personal belief or guiding principles about how they wish to eat and live and why. In order to live by a personal food philosophy, you have to take charge of specific areas of your life. You have to set goals and communicate priorities and preferences. You also have to put a strategy in place for execution to support your success.

Establishing a food philosophy is no different from committing to any other personal regimen. Consider people who have developed a longtime meditation practice. In order to establish a meaningful practice, they had to set aside time regularly to meditate and follow through with their intentions. Otherwise, a consistent meditation practice would be nothing more than wishful thinking. The same thing applies to healthier eating habits. If you don't put strategies in place to support your healthy-eating goals, optimal health for you and your family will slip through your fingers.

In this chapter, you'll begin to lay out your execution strategy to help you take steps toward attaining and sustaining the healthy-eating habits you want for yourself and your family. These steps will be based on the beliefs about food identified in Chapter 8. If you recall from Chapter 1, the key to your family crossing the finish line is dependent upon all family members practicing healthier habits consistently over time until those habits become woven into their lifestyle. Naturally, many ways exist to approach healthier eating, so creating a strategy tailored to your family's beliefs and lifestyle will ensure your success as you put your plan in motion.

You have the power and authority to make conscious choices about the way you wish to eat. As you take action to execute your own personal philosophy about your health and your eating style, you'll start to feel less like a victim in this hurried, fast-food nation and more in control. When you're crystal clear on your food preferences, you won't feel stressed each time someone offers you an indulgence you probably shouldn't have.

For example, if a co-worker brings a box of hot doughnuts by your desk, you won't need to panic. Your conviction to healthier eating minimizes the "Should I or shouldn't I eat this?" tug-of-war that commonly goes on inside our heads when we feel conflicted about eating something we know isn't good for us. Without a food philosophy, you may feel compelled to eat a doughnut just because it was offered. Now armed with clear intentions and a workable strategy, you have the power to say "no thanks." You came to work prepared to eat healthy throughout the day by bringing a container of freshly picked and washed blueberries, along with a carton of yogurt. However, if you do decide to eat a doughnut, you can choose to cut back or eliminate sugar and other highly processed foods for the remainder of the day in order to maintain a sense of balance. Learning how to handle unhealthy eating situations will help you teach your kids how to say no to foods aren't good for them.

WHAT LIFE WILL YOU CHOOSE?

All of us have to eat to live. We can't escape food. James Beard, known by many as the father of American-style gourmet cooking, poignantly captured the essence of food when he said "Food is our common ground, a universal experience." So the question before you is, "How do you want to eat?" as this decision ultimately defines how you want to *live*.

The adage "You are what you eat" is ringing true in the lives of youth and adults in this country every day. The nutritional content of the foods we eat plays a direct role in the makeup of our bodies. This is evident by the increased consumption of processed "fake" foods over the last 30 years, which has led to an epidemic of obesity and obesity-related diseases. The diagnosis of diabetes, heart disease, high blood pressure, and some cancers can mean an impaired quality of life, and in many cases death. What's most alarming is that many of those diagnosed will be children. Due to the early onset of disease for these kids, some as young as 5 years old, the negative impact such a diagnosis will have on their lives will be extensive.

When you look forward to the rest of your life, do you want to be chronically tired, stressed, overweight, and dependent on medicines to keep your blood pressure, cholesterol, and diabetes in check? Do you want to live in fear of losing your eyesight or the feeling in your hands and feet due to diabetes? I'm sure you don't want life to pass you by while you spend most of your time in waiting room chairs or on examination tables or hospital beds. And I am almost certain this isn't the kind of life you have envisioned for your child.

You have the authority and control to create a healthier, happier, and more hopeful life for you and your family. Will you exercise your authority to create the life you want, or will you hand over control of your health to chance? Will you also take responsibility for ensuring a brighter future for your child?

QUICK WINS TIPS

- Get quiet and listen to your body. It will tell you the type of food it needs.

- If you know someone who has a particular eating style, ask them in a polite, non-threatening way why they chose to eat that way. People love sharing their stories.

- Reconnect with food and cooking and enjoy the amazing ways food nourishes the body.

- Seek inspiration for the change you desire to make.

A STARTING POINT

A large body of research strongly supports that eating a healthy diet and maintaining a healthy weight, in addition to not smoking and exercising regularly, can reduce risk of the most common and deadly chronic diseases by as much as 80 percent. In other words, the quality of your life is largely determined by your fork and your feet. Dr. David Katz, director and co-founder of the Yale Prevention Research Center, describes eating and exercise habits as the "levers of medical destiny." This simply means that the diet and exercise choices you make can sway your medical outcome in the direction of health, despite the disease precursors that may lurk in your genes. Lifestyle is indeed powerful!

If you're ready to take charge, the first step is to pause and examine your beliefs and attitudes about food. This exercise will help you evaluate where your eating habits currently are and where you want to go with regard to a new eating style.

You know the saying: "If you don't know where you're going, any road will take you there." If you want to be a success, you have to be intentional about what you want. As you work through the thought process, you'll define the foods you want to eat more of, those you wish to eat less of, and those you want to avoid altogether. The result of this exercise will be your food philosophy. A food philosophy may sound grandiose, but it's basically a set of self-created intentions about how you'll eat and why. You'll find that defining your intentions and developing them into a personal philosophy will be the biggest Quick Win of all, as it will serve as the foundation for all other actions you take. Once you've created your own food philosophy, have a conversation with your family and together create a family food philosophy.

MY JOURNEY

Without much introspection, you may already know that your own belief system about food and eating needs to change if you're to have any chance at embracing a healthier eating style. No problem. You can change the way you eat any time you want to. I know because I did it.

> "A journey of a thousand miles
> begins with a single step."
> **LAO-TZU, CHINESE PHILOSOPHER**

I began my journey toward better eating habits a little differently than most people. I didn't join a weight-loss program or try one of the thousands of diet pills on the market. I didn't crash diet or rely on popular diet plans like the South Beach Diet or Atkins Diet. These approaches to weight loss weren't appealing to me because they've proved to be temporary fixes for most people. Diets are based on rules about what you can't eat. Just the word "diet" conjures up feelings of deprivation for most people. Deprivation isn't appealing to many people. That's why most diets are short lived. They simply don't represent real life and real eating habits. When people start diets, they usually have a predefined endpoint in mind. These endpoints typically revolve around a time period (I'll do the Cabbage Diet for one week), or a specific amount of weight lost (I'll do the South Beach Diet until I lose 10 pounds), or a specific clothing size (I'll do the Atkins Diet to help me drop down to a size 10). The rate of failure using these methods is astoundingly high; in fact, the Centers for Disease Control (CDC) reports the diet failure rate is 98 percent.

> **QUICK WINS TIPS**
>
> If your food philosophy supports a way of eating that includes simple recipes, ingredients, and cooking techniques, you'll be much more likely to stick with it.

Food philosophies built around more long-term lifestyle approaches to eating lead to greater opportunities for success. Individuals and families who eat and live by a particular food philosophy tend to be more self-aware of what they're eating. Adopting a particular food philosophy, like vegetarianism or sustainable eating, keeps your food habits front and center because you're continuously evaluating your meals to ensure they adhere to your principles. Some attributes of food that would be of interest to conscious eaters include the list of ingredients, nutrient content, serving size, environmental impact, and health effects.

Philosophies about food are just as varied as individuals themselves. Some people approach food as medicine. Others view their eating style as a way to take a stand against cruelty to animals and switch to a vegetarian diet. A locavore is someone who eats food primarily, if not exclusively, from their local region. As you can see, each person brings a unique perspective to food and eating; and yet, as James Beard recognized, food still serves as a common ground among us.

For my situation, instead of taking a route prone to failure, I chose a more holistic approach to eating better and maintaining a normal weight. I began by framing my belief system about food and its relevance in my own life. I explored food for what it really is—nourishment for our bodies.

CHEW ON THIS

Here are a few common food philosophies that can influence what we choose to eat:

○ *Natural food:* Eating natural means consuming unprocessed or minimally processed foods that don't contain food additives like preservatives and artificial flavorings or colors. Individuals eating this way consume foods as close as possible to their whole, unprocessed state.

○ *Raw:* Raw food hasn't been cooked or heated above 116 degrees. In raw diets, food's natural enzymes aren't altered during preparation. These enzymes have been found to aid in the body's ability to digest, absorb, and use food. Unprocessed foods are also known to have a lesser impact on blood-sugar levels than processed foods.

○ *Sustainable, seasonal, fresh, local:* These terms are used somewhat interchangeably to describe a way of eating that supports the environment, local farmers, and community connections. Sustainable growth practices include crop rotations, and grass-fed and pasture-raised animals that reduce the amount of toxic land chemicals and greenhouse gases. Eating foods that are in season, fresh, and purchased locally is good for the environment, supports local farmers, and offers the community access to quality food as well as the opportunity to know where their food comes from.

○ *Vegan:* A vegan diet is devoid of all animal products and byproducts (parts of a slaughtered animal that aren't directly consumed by humans). Thus, vegans don't eat animal flesh, dairy products or eggs, or foods made with these items.

○ *Vegetarian:* Individuals following a vegetarian lifestyle don't eat animals of any kind, including fish and shellfish. Vegetarians eat a plant-based diet, which may include dairy products such as eggs, yogurt and cheese.

As a child I learned a version of grace that has been said over meals in my family for several generations. Before our first bite, our grace was and still is, "Dear God, thank you for this food we are about to receive for the nourishment of our bodies. In the Name of Christ our Savior. Amen." This realization served as the foundation of my food philosophy. As I stated in Chapter 2, my eating style reflects my belief that food should taste good, nourish the body and preserve health. This approach to eating helped me reduce my clothing size from a women's size 12-14 to a size 6-8 and successfully keep it off for more than 12 years.

Just because you were raised to eat a certain way doesn't mean you have to eat that way all your life. You can change your eating style anytime you like. I was raised on traditional, Southern-style foods like fried chicken, cornbread and vegetables seasoned with meat. So you can imagine how challenging it was to change my habits. One part of my mind was pulling me toward attaining a healthy and fit body, while the other part was creating a dialogue focused on deprivation and fear. Some days the conflict was agonizing, but my food philosophy enabled me to reclaim control of my mind. This was critical, because thoughts lead to actions, and actions lead to habits. I didn't change my unhealthy habits all at once. Some people can quit bad habits cold turkey, but that approach wasn't for me. Instead, I quit eating fried chicken on a regular basis and only indulged in it when visiting my mom or grandma, which I did about once a month.

IT'S YOUR TURN

Explore your beliefs about food and health, the environment, and economic and social issues related to food before you commit to any diet changes. Once you commit to a choice, be prepared to defend it. You can be sure there will be many times when you'll have to defend your lifestyle choice, such as when friends ask you to go out for dessert, or co-workers invite you to lunch every day, or your family asks to uphold a weekly ritual (e.g., going out to dinner after church service). During those times, you must be crystal clear about your beliefs and convictions in order to remain empowered.

I've shared with you the things that served as a hook for me. Now it's time for you to decide what *your* motivators are. Use the "Food Philosophy Worksheet" on page 94 as your guide.

Small, meaningful changes in your diet can lead to huge improvements in your health and happiness over time. What you value is where you'll want to put your energy. In Chapter 10, I offer nine simple, quick, and practical strategies you can use to implement your food philosophy.

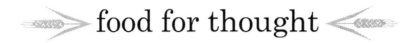

food for thought

○ Align your eating habits with your values. You'll find it will be much easier to stick to your eating plan than to eat according to someone else's values.

○ Your food philosophy will serve as an anchor to keep you firmly positioned when you feel overcome by a sea of unhealthy food choices.

FOOD PHILOSOPHY WORKSHEET

1. WHY DO YOU WANT TO CHANGE YOUR EATING STYLE?

_____

_____

_____

2. WHAT CONNECTIONS WITH FOOD, BEYOND TASTE, RESONATE WITH YOU?

_____

_____

_____

   A. DO YOU WANT TO ABSTAIN FROM THE KILLING OF ANIMALS FOR FOOD PRODUCTION?_____

   B. DO YOU BELIEVE STRONGLY IN SUPPORTING THE LOCAL ECONOMY?_____

   C. DO YOU BELIEVE IN THE POWER OF FOOD TO HEAL AND PROTECT THE BODY?_____

3. DO YOU WANT TO PROTECT THE ENVIRONMENT AND SAVE MONEY BY EATING MORE LOCAL, SEASONALLY GROWN FOODS?

_____

_____

_____

4. WHAT REALLY APPEALS TO YOU ABOUT EATING FRESHER, LESS PROCESSED FOODS?

_____

_____

_____

WRITE YOUR FOOD PHILOSOPHY:

_____

_____

_____

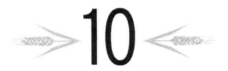

10

9 QUICK WINS

By now, you've carefully examined your family's eating habits as well as the impact of poor lifestyle choices on your health and the health of your kids. You can easily identify the habits that keep your family from eating the foods you know are best. When you eat well, you feel well. And when you consume too many processed foods and restaurant meals, your health suffers, your food budget goes through the roof, your kids' learning potential is affected, and the behaviors you're teaching your kids will set them on a course for health problems that will follow them into adulthood.

If you decide to trade in your old lifestyle, you now have the tools to make your dreams of a healthier, more vibrant life a reality. You're empowered to take charge of your life. As a parent, you're also empowered to provide a healthier lifestyle for your children.

You didn't get where you are overnight, so it's impossible to change the way your family eats all at once. You have to experiment with new foods, new ways of cooking and new eating schedules in order to transform your family's diet and, subsequently, their lives. So break them in gently.

This chapter offers nine simple steps you can take right now to help everyone start eating and living healthier. Approached consistently and systematically, these simple steps will lead to *big* changes in your family's life.

1. EAT A NOURISHING BREAKFAST EVERY DAY

Breakfast is the most important meal of the day—*really*. Eating breakfast "breaks the fast" your body has been in since the last time you ate, the night before. A nourishing breakfast is rich in nutrients, fiber, protein, and other essentials that the body recognizes as excellent sources of fuel. Breakfast replenishes depleted energy stores that become drained during the night while we sleep, and that's especially important for the brain. In fact, studies show that kids who eat breakfast perform better in school. When the body is properly fueled, kids are more focused, have stable energy levels and enjoy better moods. Eating breakfast also helps adults feel better throughout the day and perform better at work.

I know mornings are hectic times for busy families. Kids don't want to get up, spouses don't want to get up, no one knows what they want to wear to school, the dog needs to be walked, and the minutes on the clock are steadily ticking away. Skipping breakfast may seem like a smart strategy to save time in the mornings, but leaving the house without a nourishing breakfast will likely cause you and your kids to feel tired, unfocused, and drained of energy throughout the day.

A simple, quick, and nutritious breakfast will set the right tone for everyone's day and can fit into your busy morning schedule. The easiest way to for everyone in the house to start off the day is with a glass of fresh water to rehydrate the body with fluid lost during the night. It only takes a couple of seconds to grab a glass of water. A nourishing breakfast should include lean protein and fiber-rich carbohydrates that will satisfy hunger and keep everyone feeling full throughout the morning. Good protein staples include lean, high-quality meats; eggs; quinoa; beans; and low-fat dairy. Excellent fiber staples include whole grains, vegetables, and fruit. Stay away from highly processed foods like sugary cereals, white bread, instant grits and syrups, which are rapidly digested and will leave kids feeling hungry and tired before the morning even gets started.

In our house, a simple breakfast often looks like this for my husband, son, and me:

- Boiled eggs
- 100% whole-wheat toast with 1 teaspoon butter
- Fresh fruit (apple slices, bananas, grapes, blueberries or strawberries) or canned fruit in its own juice (mandarin oranges, pears or pineapples)
- 1% milk or 100% orange juice

Or

○ Bowl of whole-grain cereal like Cheerios
○ 1% milk
○ 100% whole wheat toast with 1 teaspoon butter
○ Fruit

2. EAT 5 TO 6 NOURISHING, SMALL MEALS/SNACKS PER DAY

Busy, active, healthy families don't need to eat a lot—they need to eat often! Eating several small meals throughout the day is your family's secret health weapon to achieving abundant energy, mental clarity, and a healthy weight. Simple, nourishing food spread throughout the day provides your body with clean fuel to keep it running optimally all day long. A steady supply of nutrients in the form of lean protein, healthy fats, and wholesome fruits and vegetables will keep you feeling full all day, increase your metabolism, and help you avoid cravings.

The size of your snacks and meals depends upon your caloric needs. However, a good rule of thumb for healthy snacking is to keep snacks in the 100- to 300-calorie range. Aim for healthy meals between 300 and 600 calories, including your beverage. Drinks can add a lot of calories to your daily mix, so if you want to spend your calories wisely and get the most bang for your buck, drink water or low-fat milk, and save your calories for real food.

So how do you go about eating five to six small meals a day instead of three larger ones? First, don't let the notion of eating so many times a day overwhelm you. Having access to a constant supply of nutritious food roughly every 2 to 3 hours will take a little bit of planning, but not much more than you're already doing. You probably already eat roughly three meals a day, so all you're trying to do is add two snacks: one between breakfast and lunch, and the other between lunch and dinner. You can add an extra-light snack after dinner if you need a little something before going to bed.

I've provided a sample of my eating schedule (see "Tonya's Eating Schedule" on page 98) to help you get started. Take a few moments and use the blank charts on page 98 to figure out how to space out your eating schedule so you can fit in two or three extra snacks each day. Then sit down with your spouse and kids to help them prepare an eating schedule.

TONYA'S EATING SCHEDULE

Breakfast	7:30 am
Morning Snack	10:00 am
Lunch	12:30 pm
Afternoon Snack	3:00 pm
Dinner	6:30 pm
Evening Beverage*	8:30 pm

MOM'S EATING SCHEDULE

Breakfast	
Morning Snack	
Lunch	
Afternoon Snack	
Dinner	
Evening Beverage	

KIDS' EATING SCHEDULE

Breakfast	
Morning Snack	
Lunch	
Afternoon Snack	
Dinner	
Evening Beverage	

DAD'S EATING SCHEDULE

Breakfast	
Morning Snack	
Lunch	
Afternoon Snack	
Dinner	
Evening Beverag	

* *Healthy beverage suggestions include green tea, black tea, or water with fresh fruit slices, such as cucumbers, lemons, limes, or strawberries.*

Here are some tips to help you get started:

1. *Start slowly.* Don't try to jump from eating three meals a day to six meals and snacks overnight. Look over the eating schedule you completed above and pick one snack to focus on. Take a couple of days to work that snack into your eating regimen, then focus on adding another.

2. *Rely on staples.* Do a little research to find at least five healthy snacks you and your family like and have access to. Purchase what you need, prepare it if necessary (i.e., wash, chop), and store it so it's there when you need it. Integrating planned snacks into your diet will become a no-brainer, thus eliminating the stress of constantly trying to figure out what you and your family can eat for a snack.

3. *Split meals.* Prepare what you normally eat for breakfast, but only eat half of it. Pack the other half in a storage container or baggie for you to eat later as your mid-morning snack.

QUICK WINS TIPS

Here are some great snack suggestions:

° Fruit smoothies (8-12 ounces)

° 1 mozzarella string-cheese stick

° 1 ounce chopped walnuts (14 shelled halves)

° 1 medium-sized piece of fresh fruit, such as apples, bananas, blueberries, strawberries, or oranges

° 1 cup mixed green salad with homemade oil and vinegar dressing

° 1/2 turkey sandwich on whole wheat bread

Refer back to the "Healthy Snacks" list in Chapter 3 for more ideas.

---

3. READ NUTRITION LABELS ON PACKAGED FOODS

The key to a healthier diet lies in knowing exactly what it is you're eating. So if you're about to eat a food item from a package with a nutrition label on it—read it! The foods that are best for your body, like fresh, leafy greens, tomatoes, and squash, won't have a label.

Required by the Food and Drug Administration (FDA), nutrition labels are useful tools that can help you make accurate, quick, and informed food choices. A standard label includes serving size, calories, nutrients (e.g. fat, carbohydrates, protein, vitamins, and minerals), percentage of daily value of nutrients, a footnote detailing percentage daily values of nutrients for a typical 2,000-calorie diet, and a list of ingredients in order of decreasing weight. That's a lot of good information. If you focused on processing all this information on every food package, you'd be in the grocery store a long time. So it's important for you to spend a few minutes in "Nutrition Facts Label 101" before you head out to the store.

Boosting your label-reading skills is easy. And you can start teaching your kids to be label-savvy too, when they're in elementary school. My son learned to interpret serving sizes when he was in second grade. My advice to you, in reading the nutrition label, is to focus on at least the following key elements for vital information to help you decide whether to "love it" or "leave it":

1. *Serving size:* Usually found at the top of the label, serving size indicates the size of a standard serving and how many servings the package contains based on standard measures agreed on by the U.S. Department of Agriculture and the FDA. This is where you have to be extra careful—and read that label—or you could end up consuming more than you bargained for.

2. *Calories:* Calories are a measure how of much energy you can get from food. Weight gain occurs when you consistently consume more calories than you burn. When you eat, make sure you factor in the number of calories for each serving of food you consume.

3. *Saturated fat and trans fat:* These fats should be limited or avoided in a healthy diet because they increase cholesterol levels and risk of heart disease. The American Heart Association recommends limiting daily saturated fat intake to 7 percent of your daily caloric intake. So a person on an 1,800-calorie diet should consume no more than 126 calories, or roughly 14 grams, from saturated fat. The limits for trans fat, or partially hydrogenated oils, are much lower, less than 1 percent of daily calories. Many of my clients ask me how a product can be labeled "no trans fat" but still have partially hydrogenated oil listed in the ingredients list. The label on the front of the package stating that the product doesn't contain trans fat is a marketing tool. The manufacturer is using that claim to draw you to their product. By law, if the product contains half a gram

or less of trans fats, it can bear the trans-fat-free claim. See why it pays to be label-savvy?

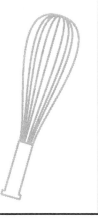

BELIEVE IT OR NOT

Sweetened applesauce can have as much as 22 grams of sugar in one cup. There's no recommended daily allowance for sugar, but it's suggested that children's daily caloric intake not exceed 10 percent.

4. *Sodium:* Sodium, or salt, content is of specific concern to people suffering or at risk for high blood pressure, a leading cause of heart disease. Healthy advice: Choose packaged foods that contain 5 percent or less of the daily value of sodium. For more information on sodium, see Chapter 8.

5. *Dietary fiber:* The amount of fiber in a product is listed under "total carbohydrates." Experts recommend consuming 25 to 38 grams of fiber a day. Keep a tally of your fiber intake and make sure you hit the mark each day to relieve constipation (especially common in children), keep your digestive system running smoothly, and manage weight. A good rule of thumb is to choose products with at least 3 to 5 grams of fiber per serving.

6. *Sugar:* Sugar is largely empty calories, offering no nutritional value. Many packaged food items like soda and candy contain added sugar to enhance taste. Other food products may contain naturally occurring sugars like fructose (fruit sugar) and lactose (milk sugar). Sugar comes in many forms and can be listed in the ingredients list by any one of the following names: sugar syrup, corn syrup, high-fructose corn syrup, juice concentrate, refiner's syrup, maltose, dextrose, sucrose, honey, and maple syrup. For more information on sugar, see Chapter 8.

7. *Ingredients:* Listed in descending order of weight from most to least, longer lists are suggestive of more processed foods, so choose foods with a very short list of recognizable ingredients. Dr. Mehmet Oz says consumers should run, not walk, if they see these five ingredients in their food: simple sugar; high-fructose corn syrup; enriched (white), bleached, or refined flour; trans fat; and hydrogenated oil.

Realage.com has a nifty interactive online food label decoder that's a great tool for helping families decipher food labels and use the information more effectively and easily to make wise food choices. The FDA website is another great resource for an extensive overview of the nutrition facts label.

4. SEEK LOCAL SOURCES OF FRESH PRODUCE AS OFTEN AS POSSIBLE

Across the country, farmer's markets and vegetable stands are popping up everywhere. If you take notice as you're driving or riding around your community, you're sure to see a farmer's market operating in a store parking lot or bustling just off the highway. The growing demand for quality local produce has given small farmers an opportunity to share their freshest harvest with the people who live near them. And what a benefit to all of us! Local produce is tastier, fresher, and more nutritious. Supporting your local farmer gives your family an opportunity to know where your food comes from. Getting to know your local farmer provides a great opportunity for you to personally teach your child how food is grown. Unfortunately, many children in this country are so accustomed to processed food that they have no awareness of what real food looks like.

By buying local you gain piece of mind, knowing your food was carefully grown and recently harvested to give you the best food product available. And when you choose to buy and eat local, you're supporting your local agriculture and doing your part to keep your family connected to good food. Plus, locally grown produce is frequently cheaper than grocery store counterparts. Locally grown organic produce is also typically cheaper at farmer's markets. Farmers can afford to charge less for their food when the cost of production is lower. No expensive transportation costs are incurred to drive the food right down the road from their farms. As a result, local farmers are able to pass their savings on to you. When your produce is fresher and cheaper at farmer's markets, how can a family go wrong?

BELIEVE IT OR NOT

During a recent television episode of *Jamie Oliver's Food Revolution,* very few elementary school kids were able to recognize basic vegetables like tomatoes or potatoes. It's time for families to get back to the basics for our children's sake.

Need more reasons to buy local? Here are six more. Local produce...

1. Tastes better
2. Is better for you
3. Is cheaper
4. Supports the environment
5. Preserves our health
6. Supports local farmers and the local economy

For tips on finding and getting the most out of farmer's markets, see our "Farmer's Market Shopping Guide" in Appendix F.

5. LIMIT FOOD CHOICES WHEN EATING OUT

Despite your family's best efforts to eat more, simple, and natural home-cooked meals, it isn't always possible. But don't panic—that doesn't mean the family's healthy eating habits have to go flying out the window whenever you choose to eat out.

One thing to remember about eating is that increased options generally lead to increased consumption. This is true for adults and for children. For this reason, one of the best ways to avoid eating too much of the wrong food is to limit your food choices. Meal descriptions on restaurant menus are designed to appeal to your senses. Kid's menus are full of puzzles, games, and fun things to color—and they're also full of calorie-loaded pizza, processed hot dogs, and french fries. The adult menus can be even worse, with extra-large portions and calorie-loaded appetizers. For example, according to the book *Eat This, Not That! for Kids!*, by David Zinczenko, Chili's Pepper Pals Country-Fried Chicken Crispers with ranch dressing and home-style fries has 1,110 calories, 82 grams of fat, and 1,980mg sodium—and qualifies as one of the worst kid's meals in America. I know my son could eat this meal in one sitting if I offered it to him, and I'll bet your elementary-school-aged children would as well.

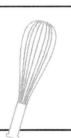

BELIEVE IT OR NOT

One serving of supersize french fries packs more than 600 calories.

As parents, we have a strong influence over the foods our kids eat. We should be diligent about steering our children toward healthy food choices and provide guidance that will enable them to soon make healthy choices their own. An occasional Pepper Pals chicken meal is OK, but if your children eat this caliber meal several times a week, you're setting them up for a lifetime of poor eating habits and the poor health consequences that may accompany them.

Familiarize yourself with restaurant menus beforehand and have a basic idea of which options you'll offer your child. Also, have a good handle on which meals you may choose for yourself. Many restaurants

BELIEVE IT OR NOT

Every day, 1 out of 4 children eat fast food.

have the nutritional content of their foods available on the web. If the restaurant doesn't have a proprietary website, you can search one of the expansive online nutritional databases like calorie-count.com, calorieking.com, or thedailyplate.com.

It's easy to select meals for your child if they haven't yet learned to read. But once they can read and interpret a restaurant menu for themselves, things can get pretty hairy. They know what they want to eat, and you could easily end up with a food fight on your hands if you don't give in to their demands.

Try these Quick Wins to cut down on calories, salt, sugar, and fat when your child is eating away from home.

○ Talk to your child before arriving at the restaurant to reiterate the importance of healthy eating habits.

○ Avoid ordering extra large portions just because they're a deal.

○ Allow your kids to order the kid's meal with healthy substitutions for fries and soda.

○ Set a good example by ordering a healthy meal yourself.

6. ESTABLISH FAMILY FOOD RULES

Some folks say rules are simply meant to be broken. I like to think of rules as a guide to encourage, support, and implement a particular behavior. When it comes to family food rules, I think they make eating easier. If you know the rules, you always know what to do, and you don't really have to think much about it.

Michael Pollan, author of *In Defense of Food* and *The Omnivore's Dilemma*, is recognized for encouraging food rules to live and eat by. Most foodies can quote his well-known food rule verbatim: "Eat food. Not too much. Mostly plants."

Food rules can actually be established to simplify many areas of your healthy eating lifestyle. For example, food rules can be implemented to help you increase variety in your diet, control food portions, establish good manners, and regulate eating out.

Food rules can be quite useful in helping children manage how to eat when they're away from home. Moderation is key to a healthy diet. Simple rules can help your children maintain balance when they're at school, at parties, with friends, or in other environments where unhealthy food may be available. How many times has your child come home and said he ate three cupcakes at a school party, or four slices of pizza at a friend's birthday party (my son did this!), or a large milkshake and a Happy Meal with Grandma? All in one week! This happens. And it's frustrating for parents who try to instill healthy eating habits at home. But what's a parent to do when their kids are "out of range"? Food rules can empower your child to make healthy choices, even when Mom and Dad are not there to guide them.

QUICK WINS TIPS

For family food rules to be effective, they should follow three basic criteria: *They should be simple, effectively communicated, and not too restrictive.*

7. CHOOSE NATURAL FOODS OVER HIGHLY PROCESSED FOODS

Whole food. Real food. Green food. Clean food. Natural food. How's a person supposed to know what to eat?

There's a growing interest in good food. As a result, a lot of widely used food terminology has been created to describe it. Each takes a slightly different approach to food, but ultimately each eating style is rooted in wholesome, nutritious, and better-for-you staples. Highly refined, processed foods don't have a place in either of these eating patterns.

FAMILY FOOD RULES STARTER LIST

Here are 20 examples of family food rules I gathered that you can use as a guide to help you create your own Family Food Rules.

1. Buy 80 percent of your groceries from the perimeter of the supermarket where the freshest food is.

2. Avoid eating any processed food item that has more than five ingredients listed on the nutrition label.

3. Avoid eating any processed food item containing high-fructose corn syrup.

4. Always choose fresh over processed.

5. Eat only one sweet treat per day.

6. Don't eat any more than [*X number* based on individual] slices of pizza at one sitting. Fill up on salad or fruit.

7. Only drink water or milk with sweet treats.

8. Eat only at the table to promote mindful eating.

9. Avoid eating any processed food item containing trans fat.

10. Eat at least three different colored fruits and vegetables each day. Maintain a journal to keep track. (See Appendix B for a sample food journal.)

11. Turn off the TV, radio and computer during meal time.

12. Eat a nourishing breakfast every day.

13. Eat a simple mixed green salad with a few fresh vegetables or fruits with dinner every night.

14. Start each day with a glass of fresh, clean water.

15. Balance splurges with smart food choices the rest of the day.

16. Take a courtesy bite of new foods before deciding you don't want them.

17. Enjoy dessert in moderation.

18. Make half of your grains whole.

19. Eat 5 to 6 small meals each day.

20. Drink a glass of water before dinner.

Here's a quick general guide to good food terms:

TERM	WHAT IT MEANS
Natural foods	Minimally processed, do not contain any additives such as preservatives, artificial colorings, flavorings, or sweeteners
Organic foods	Crops and livestock grown without synthetic chemicals, antibiotics, or hormones
Whole foods	Unprocessed, unrefined, or as close to original state as possible
Green foods	Organically produced, local, seasonal food
Clean foods	Foods free of artificial preservatives, coloring, irradiation, synthetic pesticides, fungicides, ripening agents, fumigants, drug residues and growth hormones

Although you know that foods as close to their natural state as possible are better for you than highly processed foods, getting your family on board is an entirely different story. Food marketing and peer pressure make processed food more appealing. Kids want what other kids are eating, and for most kids in America that equates to pizza, processed meats, fries, Pop Tarts, and other calorie-dense foods. As a parent, you're responsible for ensuring your kids eat nutritiously, but at the same time you don't want to be seen as the food police. Coax your kids into eating more natural foods. Set food rules that establish family expectations for healthful eating habits. Make sure that an appealing and deliciously prepared vegetable is always offered at dinner time. Kids don't want mushy vegetables or vegetables with strong seasonings. Offer them lightly steamed, cruciferous vegetables like broccoli or cauliflower. For younger kids, give their vegetables funny names. When my son was in preschool, my husband and I called broccoli "trees." The rule was that each time "trees" were served, he didn't have to eat them all, but he did have to eat at least one of them. My husband and I were consistent with this food rule, and soon my son learned that was our expectation, and he ate his tree without a lot of protest.

8. USE SMALL PLATES/SMALL PORTIONS

A few months ago, I started eating on salad plates like the ones my son eats on—you know, the typical 9-inch plates that come in standard sets of dinner plates and coffee mugs. I wanted to see if I could reduce my portions sizes without really missing the extra food that wasn't on my plate. In the past, I've tried preparing a normal plate of food and leaving 25 percent on my plate. That strategy didn't work too well for me because in the back of my mind I viewed it as being wasteful. But surprisingly, I got used to eating on smaller plates rather quickly, and I was able to cut back on my portion sizes without much effort.

Serving dinner on smaller plates is an effective way to help your family eat less. Smaller plates trick your mind into thinking you're eating your normal-size portion of food when you're actually eating less than usual. Participants using large bowls in the study *Ice Cream Illusions: Bowls, Spoons,* and *Self-Served Portions* (published in the *American Journal of Preventive Medicine*) ate 30 percent more than participants in the study who used smaller bowls. Since people tend to eat most of what they're served, imagine how much more food people eat when they grab straight from a bag of chips or a box of cookies!

> **BELIEVE IT OR NOT**
> Individuals are subject to "portion distortion" when they perceive large portion sizes as appropriate amounts to eat at a single-eating occasion.

Try instituting smaller portions with your family. Encourage your family to pour individual servings of healthy snacks into small bowls or plates. Individual-size servings can be useful in helping your children learn to recognize sensible portions. It's hard for them to gauge how much they're eating if they're stuffing their faces straight from the bag. Plus, I think it is just good old-fashioned manners to pour snacks onto a napkin or bowl rather than digging your hands into a bag or bowl that other people are sharing. If it makes more sense economically to buy snacks in bulk, repackage individual portions in small plastic bags before making them available to your family.

Purchase a pack of 4- to 6-ounce plastic cups, and use them for drinking beverages other than water. Treat water as a special beverage and allow kids to drink it from a larger glass. Believe me, kids will notice the smaller cups you introduce faster than they'll notice the smaller plates. You'll need to establish how you'll address beverage refills other than water. In our household, we encourage the rule of only one refill of beverages other than water.

water mark

Do you encourage your kids to keep track of how much water they drink each day? Teach them how to keep a simple log. Use an index card, draw six to eight square boxes, and have your child place a check mark for each glass of water they drink.

When they reach their goal – eight glasses – reward them with stickers, a ball, special privileges, or their favorite nonfood item.

9. COOK AND EAT MORE NATURAL FOODS AT HOME

We're all creatures of habit. Once we settle into our routine of doing things a certain way, it's often hard for us to change. Whether it's driving a certain route to work, styling our hair in a particular way, or eating out instead of cooking, we tend to resist change. Think about the slight tension that rises in you when you see road construction ahead and are forced to take a detour. How does your young child react when his bedtime routine is altered the slightest bit? What each of you feels is called stress. When we get used to doing the same things day in and day out, introducing change ignites stress. Some people accept the change in stride and move on. Others resist with kicking and screaming.

Our eating habits are especially hard to change. Food is such an important element of who we are as families that when Mr. Change starts snooping around our plates, we stress out. But eating meals prepared at home is good for our diets and for our family. Home-cooked food offers better nutritional value compared to restaurant and highly processed meals. Fresh, whole, natural foods are higher in antioxidants, nutrients and fiber, and devoid of additives, such as preservatives and artificial colorings. Foods prepared at home are also typically lower in calories, salt, sugar and sodium.

Cooking at home gives you more control over the choice and quality of ingredients used to prepare meals. You're much more likely to select unblemished, pure, safe foodstuffs than some guy behind the counter who doesn't know you. I believe that the best foods are prepared by people we know, like and trust. Mom, Dad, Grandma, aunties, family, friends, et al., have our best interest at heart, not profit.

Meals cooked at home also provide increased opportunity for food variety. Food variety means eating an assortment of food with different nutrients from each of the five food groups on a consistent basis. Variety is important because different foods provide varying amounts of nutrients. Eating a diverse diet across and within the food groups keeps meals interesting, which, by the way, is critical if you want to get your family onboard with eating healthier. Variety also improves the quality of your diet. Most of the variety in your diet should come from plants. Food variety also helps prevent chronic diseases, such as heart disease, diabetes and some cancers.

Cooking and preparing meals at home not only saves your health, but it also saves you money. Compare the cost of meals you cook at home to dining out. You can buy a basket of groceries for the price of feeding a family of four at a chain restaurant.

It's very easy to shake up your routine and make room for some new and interesting home cooked foods. Here are some suggestions:

○ *Plan weekly menus with grocery shopping lists.* Make sure meals complement each other so leftovers can be paired with new meals to keep boredom and food waste at a minimum.

○ *Make sure Family Food Rules specify the number of meals eaten at home each week.* See the "Family Food Rules Starter List" on page 106.

○ *Experiment with a new vegetable each week.* Make a list of the ones you tried so you don't revert back to old favorites out of habit.

○ *Experiment with new cooking methods.* Try roasting, steaming, sautéing, boiling, grilling or braising vegetables.

○ *Make meat a side item instead of the main course so you can make room for a new whole grain.* Some of my favorites are couscous, quinoa, barley and brown rice.

○ *Make pizza at home using fresh vegetables and cheeses instead of ordering takeout.* Get everyone involved for a fun family activity and a nourishing experience.

food for thought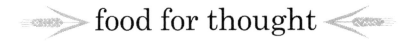

- ○ The Quick Wins provided in this chapter are offered to serve as a starting point for your new, healthier habits. Review the entire list carefully. Then choose one simple step to start first. Once you and your family have begun practicing the new habit at least 80 percent of the time, add on another Quick Win!

- ○ Once you add on a new Quick Win, remember not to abandon the previous healthy habits you've adopted. Building a lifestyle of healthy eating is a cumulative process.

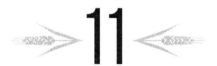

TO YOUR HEALTH

Once I really "got" the connection between my food and my health, my life changed. I became an ally with my food in the pursuit of a healthier and happier life. My new empowered relationship supported a strong conviction to feed my body as well as I could, when I could, in order to preserve my health for as long as possible. I have a young son, and I want to instill a legacy of optimal health for his future. I also want to continue a life of optimal health so I can enjoy my son in his adult years, and eventually enjoy being a vibrant and loving grandmother to his future children.

I've watched the elders in my family battle weight issues and chronic disease for years. One by one, I'm beginning to see the younger generation of my family, my cousins, succumbing to weight gain and putting themselves at risk for the related illnesses that accompany added pounds. One cousin has developed diabetes. An aunt has, too. My grandmother died of cancer. My grandfather passed away suddenly of a heart attack. This isn't the legacy I want for my son, or any other child in this country.

As a result of seeing the effects of obesity and poor health up close, I made a personal choice to change my relationship with food. I am empowered every day to approach food and eating with balance. If I overindulge, I cut back later. Each and every time I get off track with my healthy eating habits, I'm aware, and I get back on track. There was a popular Christian song by Donnie McClurkin with lyrics that speak of our imperfect human nature and our blessed opportunity to get back up after we've fallen down. And a proverb from the *Holy Bible* says that a righteous man falls seven times and gets up each time.

> "Eating is not merely a material pleasure.
> Eating well gives a spectacular joy to life and
> contributes immensely to goodwill and happy
> companionship. It is of great importance to the morale."
> **ELSA SCHIAPARELLI**

The one thing that's most different about me now, compared to 16 years ago, is that I'm attracted to food for more than just its taste. I connect with food on a much deeper level. I'm grateful for the health-promoting power of natural food. I understand the many ways that good food speaks to the soul. I see how food connects and divides people. I understand the influence food has on the legacy of my family. Your family may not always be able to choose the best foods. Perhaps you or your spouse has been laid off and money is extremely tight in your household right now. Maybe you live in an area designated as a "food desert"—an area of the country with little or no access to grocery stores that offer high-quality produce or other natural foods necessary to maintain a healthy diet. Whatever your situation, there are always ways—even if it's just switching from soda to water at meal times—to make a healthier choice.

That's what healthy living is all about. Awareness, knowledge, and balance.

My best to you. May you love your family to *life!*

notes

APPENDIX A
MY QUICK WINS HEALTH JOURNAL

The Quick Wins Health Journal is about taking charge of your health and your lifestyle. Maintaining healthy habits and monitoring your health information will dictate the quality of your health. This journal is designed to help you keep track of your weight, blood pressure, lab results, family history, and other vital information to help you and your family live healthier.

Start to fill in this journal *now*. Check with your doctor and family members for any information you don't know. Review your Quick Wins Health Journal weekly, monthly, or as often as necessary to stay in tune with your health status and to keep a check on health issues that are of concern to you and your family. This journal is also a great way to keep track of your health goals and any questions you have for your physician.

NAME_____

MY THOUGHTS ABOUT MY HEALTH:

_____

_____

_____

_____

MY THOUGHTS ABOUT MY FAMILY'S HEALTH:

_____

_____

_____

_____

DATE OF MOST RECENT PHYSICAL EXAM: _____

HEIGHT:

Date: _____feet: _____inches: _____

WEIGHT:

Date: _____ lbs/kg: _____

Date: _____ lbs/kg: _____

Date: _____ lbs/kg: _____

BLOOD PRESSURE:

Date: _____ systolic: _____ diastolic: _____

Date: _____ systolic: _____ diastolic: _____

Date: _____ systolic: _____ diastolic: _____

CHOLESTEROL:

Date: _____ Total cholesterol: _____ LDL ("bad"): _____ HDL ("good"): _____

Date: _____ Total cholesterol: _____ LDL ("bad"): _____ HDL ("good"): _____

Date: _____ Total cholesterol: _____ LDL ("bad"): _____ HDL ("good"): _____

DIABETES (BLOOD SUGAR):

Date: _____Fasting Blood Glucose Result: _____mg/dl

Date: _____Post-meal (Postprandial) Blood Glucose Result: _____mg/dl

MY FAMILY'S CHRONIC HEALTH HISTORY:

RELATIONSHIP	CHRONIC ILLNESS
MOTHER	
FATHER	
BROTHER(S)	
SISTER(S)	
MATERNAL GRANDMOTHER	
MATERNAL GRANDFATHER	
PATERNAL GRANDMOTHER	
PATERNAL GRANDFATHER	
CHILD	
CHILD	
CHILD	

MY QUESTIONS ABOUT MY HEALTH:

1. _____
2. _____
3. _____
4. _____

THE ONE THING I WANT TO CHANGE MOST ABOUT MY HEALTH IS:

_____
_____
_____
_____

ONE GOOD THING THAT WOULD HAPPEN IF I MADE THIS CHANGE IS:

_____

_____

_____

_____

**THE ONE THING THAT IS STOPPING ME OR MAKING IT
SO HARD FOR ME TO CHANGE IS:**

_____

_____

_____

_____

THE ONE THING I KNOW I CAN DO TO OVERCOME THIS OBSTACLE IS:

_____

_____

_____

_____

APPENDIX B
MY QUICK WINS DAILY FOOD JOURNAL

NAME _____ **DATE:** _____

FOOD GROUP	FOOD NAME	AMOUNT
Breakfast		
Grains		
Vegetables		
Fruits		
Dairy		
Protein		
Fats		
Beverages		
Sweets		
Snack		
Notes		
Lunch		
Grains		
Vegetables		
Fruits		
Dairy		
Protein		
Fats		
Beverages		
Sweets		
Snack		
Notes		
Dinner		
Grains		
Vegetables		
Fruits		
Dairy		
Protein		
Fats		
Beverages		
Sweets		
Snack		
Notes		

Water (8 glasses) ❑ ❑ ❑ ❑ ❑ ❑ ❑ ❑

APPENDIX C
QUICK WINS LOG

Use this log to chronicle your journey to a healthier way of eating. Take note of the things you experience along the way, like a boost in your energy level or a new food your child was willing to try. Use our Quick Wins Log or create your own!

DATE	ACTION TAKEN	RESULT

APPENDIX D
QUICK WINS HEALTHY ESSENTIALS

ESSENTIAL COOKING TOOLS CHECKLIST:
7 KITCHEN TOOLS TO INSPIRE HEALTHY EATING

The healthiest meals are the ones you cook at home. You can make cooking healthy meals quick and easy with the right equipment. I'm always looking for new ways to be inspired to cook. When I'm running low on energy and motivation, some of my favorite cooking tools help make the job easier and family time around the dinner table more rewarding.

Here's a list of 7 essential kitchen tools to inspire you to cook healthy nourishing meals for yourself and your family!

1. QUALITY CHEF'S KNIFE

Nothing feels better in your hands and makes you feel like a "real" cook than a good chef's knife. A chef's knife can be used to cut just about anything you need while cooking. The knife you choose should have a very strong, sharp blade and should feel great when gripped in your hands. According to Cooking.com's Best of Top Rated Chef's Knives, the 8-inch knife by Wusthoff was top rated in the Chef's Knife category.

2. OIL SPRAYER/MISTER

Fill your sprayer/mister with your favorite cooking oil (canola, olive oil, sesame) and use it to coat pans to prevent sticking. The benefit of these sprayers is that they will help you use less oil and they are aerosol free.

3. MULTI-CHOPPER/SLICER

This is one tool I can't live without. My brother gave it to me as a birthday present. A food chopper/slicer allows cooks to chop, dice, slice and julienne a variety of fruits and vegetables in one swift motion. They make food prep and cleanup easy and convenient. Most choppers have a catch container that allows food to be easily dumped into soups, salads, or wherever you want. These gadgets are really a life saver in the kitchen when you have lots of produce to prepare.

4. WIRE WHISK

Don't let a plain old spoon try to do the job destined for a sturdy whisk. I remember my mom using a whisk to make Southern homemade classics like gravies and thick sauces, but as I have grown into my own style of cooking, I've learned to rely on my wire whisk for many other common dishes. A sturdy whisk consisting of a long, solid handle with a series of thin wire loops joined at the end can mean the difference between lumpy pancakes or oatmeal and a breakfast that's sure to be a crowd pleaser. You may also like using a whisk to beat eggs for perfect scrambled eggs and omelets or to blend homemade cake batters.

5. CAST IRON SKILLET

Once you get over how heavy cast iron skillets are, you'll admit that every kitchen should have one. Cast iron skillets can be used to cook just about anything. They're excellent heat conductors and make food taste great. Cast iron is inexpensive and extremely durable. If your skillet hits the floor (especially a 12-inch skillet), the floor will likely crack before the skillet does. There's a myth that cast iron is hard to clean, but that's not true. Cast iron is a natural nonstick surface created by a process called seasoning. To season your pan, use a paper towel or cotton cloth to rub the entire surface with oil, such as canola, sunflower or coconut. Next, heat the pan, face down, in a 500-degree oven for 30 to 60 minutes. Once the pan cools to room temperature, the process should be repeated again. You'll know it's time to reseason your pan when food starts to stick to the surface. I have two cast iron skillets—a 10- and 12-inch. Next on my wish list is a cast iron griddle!

6. SALAD SPINNER

If you eat a lot of leafy greens at home (which I hope you do since they're so nutritious), you'll definitely want to invest in a salad spinner. I had a cheap spinner once, and it leaked and slid all across the counter every time I tried to use it. Needless to say, it ended up in the trash can. So invest in a good spinner, like an OXO Softworks brand or Kitchen Aid, to make washing greens quick and easy.

All you have to do is wash your greens, shake off excess water, fill the basket, cover with lid, and simply press an easy-to-grasp knob on top to start the basket spinning. Spin-dry greens with one hand and stop when you're ready with the built-in brake. A nonslip ring on the bottom of the spinner keeps the unit from sliding across the counter once you start spinning. Most spinners are top-rack dishwasher safe.

7. STAINLESS STEEL COOKING UTENSILS

I love the confidence I gain from using high-quality stainless steel utensils in the kitchen. I know I'm using tools that are strong enough to stir, flip, or dip anything I need. It's easy to find stainless steel slotted spoons, ladles, spatulas and spoons in longer lengths, which make them great tools for use in tall stock pots and Dutch ovens. The sturdiness of stainless steel gives cooks a sense of security when stirring, flipping or dipping hot items on the stove. It only takes one time to drop a piece of chicken back in the stockpot and have broth splash all over your blouse for you to become a convert of more durable cooking utensils.

HEALTHY PANTRY CHECKLIST

I really like pantry checklists. They're essential to smart shopping and healthy cooking. A thorough checklist helps me have a good handle on what's in my pantry and what's not, so I can save time and money while shopping and preparing nutritious meals for me and my family.

The Quick Wins Healthy Pantry Checklist is designed to help you establish a good base of healthy, nutritious pantry staples. Some of the items may be new to you. These are simple items to help you add a bit of variety to your diet. When your pantry is well-stocked, you'll find it is much easier to whip up an easy, delicious, and nutritious everyday meal in a short amount of time.

Print this list, and then pay your pantry a visit to see what you already have on hand and what you need to pick up on your next visit to the farmer's market or grocery store. You may want to consider laminating this list to make it durable—you'll be using it a lot!

WHOLE GRAINS

jasmine rice	basmati rice	brown rice	arborio rice	wild rice
whole wheat couscous	whole wheat pastas	buckwheat noodles	corn meal	polenta
quinoa	millet	bulgur	barley	oat groats
wheat berries	popcorn	buckwheat pancake mix	whole wheat breads	whole wheat tortillas
corn tortillas	rolled oats	steel-cut oats		

DRIED LEGUMES (BEANS)

lentils	red kidney beans	cannellini beans	chickpeas (garbanzo beans)	black-eyed peas
adzuki beans	five-bean mix	borlotti beans	black beans	great northern beans
pinto beans	lima beans	navy beans	split peas	

DRIED HERBS AND SPICES

curry powder	ground cumin	chili flakes	ground cinnamon	cinnamon sticks
garlic	chili powder	crushed red pepper	Italian seasoning blend	tarragon leaves
ground ginger	paprika	turmeric	seasoning blends (e.g., Mrs. Dash)	cayenne pepper
iodized salt	sea salt	kosher salt	black pepper	white pepper
nutmeg	bay leaves	basil	oregano	parsley
rosemary	thyme	cloves	allspice	sage
whole peppercorns	bouillon (beef, chicken, vegetable)	cardamom	sun-dried tomatoes	lemon pepper
dill	curry powder			

DRIED FRUITS, NUTS AND SEEDS

raisins	apricots	figs	dates	cranberries
prunes	trail mix	almonds	peanuts	brazil nuts
walnuts	pecans	mixed nuts	raw hazelnuts	raw cashews
sunflower seeds	soy nuts	sesame seeds	pumpkin seeds	

FRESH PRODUCE

potatoes	onions	shallots	garlic	lemons
root ginger	sweet potatoes	yams	tomatoes	beans

BAKING NEEDS

whole wheat flour	corn flour	all-purpose flour	whole-wheat pastry flour	breadcrumbs
quick-rising yeast	cornstarch	wheat bran	wheat germ	rolled oats
skim milk powder	dry nonfat milk	baking powder	baking soda	apple puree
yeast	baking chocolate	cornmeal	vanilla extract	lemon extract
almond extract	semisweet chocolate	cocoa		

SWEETENERS

white sugar	brown sugar	honey	powdered sugar
molasses	turbinado	agave nectar	maple syrup

OILS* AND VINEGARS

canola oil	extra virgin olive oil	peanut oil	flaxseed oil	macadamia oil
walnut oil	dark sesame oil	avocado oil	rice vinegar	distilled vinegar
malt vinegar	balsamic vinegar	cider vinegar	white wine vinegar	sherry vinegar
red wine vinegar				

use a spray or mister to reduce the amount of oil used

SAUCES AND CONDIMENTS

tomato sauce	sweet chili sauce	Worcestershire sauce	low-sodium soy sauce	prepared pesto
fish sauce	hoisin sauce	oyster sauce	hot sauce	barbecue sauce
reduced-fat mayonnaise	salsa	ketchup	dijon mustard	yellow mustard
Tabasco	horseradish	hot sauce		

SPREADS

yeast spread	honey	peanut butter (natural)	marmalade	chutneys
nut butters	all-fruit spread			

CEREALS (HOT AND COLD)

Cheerios (original)	Grape Nuts	shredded wheat	raisin bran	Total
Wheaties	wheat germ	granola bars	granola or muesli	oat bran
steel-cut oatmeal				

CANNED GOODS AND BOTTLED ITEMS

tuna	salmon	crabmeat	minced clams	chili beans
baked beans	tomatoes	tomato paste	tomato juice	curry paste
condensed milk	tomato sauce	vegetable broth	chicken broth	beef broth
light evaporated milk	coconut milk	canned fruit	corn	sweet peas
green beans	black beans	chickpeas	roasted red peppers	olives
mushrooms	chilies	artichoke hearts	kidney beans	soups
lentils	chickpeas	cannellini beans	pinto beans	pasta sauce
pineapples	peaches	fruit cocktail	mandarin oranges	tropical fruit mix
capers	chili paste	chipotle chilies in adobo sauce		

DRINKS

black tea	tea bags	herbal tea	coffee
green tea	seltzer water	water	

HEALTHY REFRIGERATOR/FREEZER CHECKLIST

In addition to a well-stocked pantry, you must also have some basic essentials in your refrigerator to make cooking at home quick and simple. You don't have to stock all these items at one time, but you'll likely find yourself relying on them frequently in your day-to-day cooking (unless you're vegan). You can find these staples at your local farmer's market, grocer, or natural-foods store.

❏ 1% or skim organic milk

❏ 100% fruit or vegetable juice

❏ Almond milk

❏ Beef (free range)—ground, roasts, steaks, tenderloin

❏ Butter

❏ Capers (optional)

❏ Cheeses—2% cheddar, feta, freshly grated parmesan, mozzarella, romano, and blue cheese

❏ Chicken breasts—boneless, skinless

❏ Chicken (free range)—whole, skinless parts, rotisserie

❏ Chicken stock (homemade if possible)

❏ Cottage cheese

❏ Cream cheese

❏ Deli meats (nitrate and nitrite free)—turkey, chicken

❏ Eggs (free range)

❏ Fresh ginger

❏ Fresh fruit—organic apples, bananas, oranges, kiwi

- ❑ Fresh produce—tomatoes, onions, peppers, herbs, lemons, limes, oranges

- ❑ Frozen cheese ravioli or tortellini

- ❑ Frozen yogurt and/or sorbet

- ❑ Fruit—peaches, blueberries, strawberries, raspberries

- ❑ Greek yogurt

- ❑ Hummus

- ❑ Keifer

- ❑ Leafy greens—spinach, kale, swiss chard, collards

- ❑ Natural peanut butter (stir and store)

- ❑ Nuts—almonds, walnuts, pine nuts, pecans

- ❑ Olives—black, green, kalamata, nicoise

- ❑ Polenta

- ❑ Reduced-fat sour cream

- ❑ Seafood—salmon, tilapia, shrimp

- ❑ Soy milk

- ❑ Soy products—tofu (soft, firm, extra firm, silken), veggie burgers, breakfast links, tempeh

- ❑ Vegetables—edamame (soybeans), broccoli, corn, bell-pepper-and-onion mix, peas, tomatoes, celery, carrots, squash, and other family favorites

- ❑ Water

- ❑ Whole grain bread, tortillas, wraps, buns

HERE'S WHAT YOU TOSS

Consider the staples in your pantry, refrigerator and freezer a health inventory. These checklists are tools to help you maintain the basics so you can whip up a quick, nutritious home-cooked meal anytime. Now that you're all stocked, carefully monitor the quality of your staples and be sure to throw away:

- Expired foods

- Highly processed foods with lots of additives

- Dented cans

- Foods containing trans fat

- High-sodium foods (daily allowance is about 2,300mg)

- High-sugar foods

5-DAY KIDS' LUNCH IDEAS

Kids need a good dose of nutritious food to keep them energized and prepared for learning throughout the day, whether they're in school, at camp, or hanging out at home.

Don't be stumped with what to put in your kids' lunchboxes. Here are some lunch suggestions to keep your kids healthy and happy. If at first your children don't like a particular item, encourage a courtesy bite of everything in their lunch tote. Offer a specific healthy food several times before abandoning it. Once they try it a couple times in a variety of ways, they might like it!

Monday	Tuna sandwich on whole wheat bread* Sliced cucumbers with low-fat ranch dressing Sliced melons, strawberries, grapes Organic milk box
Tuesday	Chicken salad sandwich on whole wheat with lettuce and tomato Leftover grilled vegetables Fruit smoothie (thermos)
Wednesday	Baked potato with black beans on the side Mixed green side salad Low-fat cream cheese with whole-wheat crackers Bottled water
Thursday	Peanut butter and jelly sandwich on whole wheat* Homemade vegetable soup (thermos) Banana 100% orange juice box
Friday	Turkey** sandwich rolled on whole wheat wrap* Pasta salad with seasonal veggies Greek yogurt with fresh blueberries Soy milk box

* Whole-wheat bread options include whole-wheat pita pockets, sliced bread, bagels, crackers, English muffins, tortillas, flatbread, or rolls.

** Use nitrate-free and nitrite-free deli meat or use home-cooked turkey.

APPENDIX E
HEALTHY-LIVING RESOURCES

COOKBOOKS TO INSPIRE YOU

I hope you're ready to get back to the basics and begin cooking simple family meals at home. I believe in starting simple, so I see no need for you to run out and get a trunk full of cookbooks and other cooking resources that will simply overwhelm you.

If you need ideas for delicious, healthy meals made with natural ingredients, I recommend you check out the titles below to get a quick grasp of great recipes, cooking and nutrition tips, and, in some cases, a brief history about good food.

Cooking Ingredients: A Practical Guide to Choosing and Using World Foods (Southwater), by Christine Ingram

Cooking Ingredients is one of my favorite cooking reference books. I rely on it at least once a week to figure out what a particular fruit or vegetable looks like, when it grows and how to prepare it. This practical guide serves as a handy reference to almost any staple a cook will need. What I really like about the current edition of this book is the true-to-life photographs, which are helpful in determining unfamiliar ingredients. The ingredients are simply categorized and thoroughly portrayed for ease of use.

The Eat-Clean Diet for Family & Kids: Simple Strategies for Lasting Health & Fitness (Robert Kennedy Publishing), by Tosca Reno

"Clean eating" is a relatively new term, but the principles behind the concept are ancient. Tosca Reno and other clean-eating converts advocate for eating whole, minimally processed food prepared without chemicals and preservatives. In other words, natural food with clean, vibrant flavors like the generations before us enjoyed. *The Eat-Clean Diet* presents practical strategies, tips, and personal anecdotes to help families get the junk out of their diets and start living a life of vibrant energy and good health. Most important, Tosca helps reassure parents that their families can eat differently and take back their lives. This book is full of great recipes with beautifully colored photographs and kid/kitchen-friendly glossy pages that will withstand accidents.

How to Cook Everything Vegetarian: Simple Meatless Recipes for Great Food (Wiley), by Mark Bittman

If you want to move gently into eating more meatless meals, this cookbook is a great place to start. The author, Mark Bittman, is brilliant at taking the scariness out of meatless meals and transforms vegetarian cuisine into family-friendly feasts. The recipes are straightforward and simple, which is refreshing to both new and busy cooks. This cookbook is huge compared with the others on this list and may seem intimidating at first glance, but you'll find it hard to resist adding it to your list of keepers.

Italian Classics (America's Test Kitchen), by the Editors of *Cook's Illustrated* Magazine

This is a foolproof collection of recipes. Each and every recipe has been "exhaustively tested" in America's Test Kitchen to find the best version. The cookbook lacks colorful photos, but the confidence you'll have going into preparing any one of the recipes from this cookbook will outweigh any need for visual reassurance. The goal of book is to provide cooks with the best techniques to transform them into better cooks. And for me, that's enough.

The Mediterranean Diet Cookbook: A Delicious Alternative for Lifelong Health (Bantam), by Nancy Harmon Jenkins

This is way more than a cookbook. Nancy Harmon Jenkins provides readers with a rich introduction to the one of the world's healthiest diets, The Mediterranean Diet. Much more than a diet, the Mediterranean way of eating is simple, delicious, and nutritious, which makes it a perfect eating style for families. This cookbook highlights foods of the Mediterranean and inspires readers to make room for good food in their lives and in our families.

Real Simple *Meals Made Easy: Quick and Simple Recipes for Every Night of the Week* (Real Simple), by the Editors of *Real Simple* Magazine

This cookbook captures all my cookbook likes between two hardback covers. The cookbook has a nice feel in my hands, the recipes are simple and practical with familiar ingredients, and they're accompanied by short and simple preparations. *Real Simple* includes a compilation of one-pot meals, no-shop meals, 30-minute meals, and freezer meals to meet the needs of today's busy cooks. There is one recipe per page, which keeps me from suffering information overload, accompanied by a full page of beautifully photographed dishes. One of the things I really appreciate about this cookbook is the tip index at the back of the book—really helpful! And lastly, this book is very affordable—under $20 at most bookstores.

Super Natural Cooking: Five Delicious Ways to Incorporate Whole and Natural Foods Into Your Cooking (Celestial Arts), by Heidi Swanson

What I love most about this cookbook are the eloquent ways Heidi describes the art of natural cooking. She has a lovely way of making natural foods feel like a special treat. This book provides a detailed introduction to whole foods and the preparation of natural ingredients. I find this book to be highly educational and a must-have for both novice and seasoned cooks.

FOOD/COOKING-RELATED WEBSITES

As with cookbooks, I believe in the adage, "keep it simple." Here are the on-line resources I rely on most for cooking healthy meals.

Allrecipes.com

A source of more than 40,000 free recipes, all created, tested, reviewed and approved by home cooks like us.

Center for Science in the Public Interest (www.cspinet.org)

Scientific information on nutrition and health, food safety and alcohol policy. The center also publishes the informative and scientifically based *Nutrition Action Healthletter*.

Eat Well Guide (www.eatwellguide.org)

A searchable database for locating local, sustainable, and organic food, no matter where you are. Search by keywords, ZIP code, or city/state to find good food near you.

Epicurious.com

A recipe website with a compilation of recipes from heavy-hitters like *Bon Appétit* and *Gourmet* magazines. The site has a database where you can store recipes you want to keep.

Local Harvest (www.localharvest.org)

A website where you can find information on farmer's markets, family farms, and other sources of fresh, local produce in your area.

National Farmer's Market Directory (http://apps.ams.usda.gov/FarmersMarkets)

A website maintained by the U.S. Department of Agriculture, offering resources on farmer's markets and local food marketing.

A FEW GREAT FOOD BLOGS

I turn to food blogs for new recipes, a fresh twist on old favorites, information, conversations with other foodies, and—most of all—inspiration.

101 Cookbooks (www.101cookbooks.com)

101 Cookbooks is the personal food journal of Heidi Swanson, author of *Super Natural Cooking*. The blog is built on her premise that if you own more than 100 cookbooks, you should start cooking—and that's what she did. Just like her cookbook, her blog is inviting and does great justice to the art of natural cooking and eating. Recipes on this site focus primarily on natural, whole foods and ingredients.

The Nourishing Gourmet (www.thenourishinggourmet.com)

The Nourishing Gourmet is a personal food blog dedicated to nourishing food. This blog is a great resource for learning how to cook healthy, natural foods on a budget. The site also includes diary and gluten-free recipes.

Raise Healthy Eaters (www.raisehealthyeaters.com)

This colorful, friendly, and inviting blog is dedicated to being a quality resource for parents who are looking for credible nutrition advice. Written by a registered dietician, this site helps parents figure out the "what" and "how" of feeding kids healthfully.

Simply Recipes (www.simplyrecipes.com)

This personal blog, created by Elise Bauer contains a few hundred recipes. What's unique about Simply Recipes is that all the recipes listed on the site have been tested by Elise or her friends and family. Thus far, every recipe I've tried has been fabulous.

APPENDIX F

FARMER'S MARKET SHOPPING GUIDE

Fresh, natural food is best for optimal health. Fortunately, there are two quick, fun and affordable ways for health-conscious families to shop for fresh produce. These include local Community Supported Agriculture (CSA) programs and farmer's markets. If you've never heard of a CSA or visited a farmer's market, now's the time. The hallmark of each of these programs is that they provide an opportunity for direct exchange of produce between the farmer and the consumer—no middleman, no scanning of barcodes and coupons. Tapping into one or both of these resources in your local area will ensure you're connected to a variety of high-quality fruits, vegetables, dairy, meats and breads.

WHAT IS A CSA PROGRAM?

CSA programs are an easy way for consumers to buy fresh, seasonal, local produce directly from farmers. As the public becomes increasingly concerned with the quality of their food, the growth of CSAs has risen dramatically over the past several years. The government doesn't track CSAs, but according to the LocalHarvest.org database, which is the most comprehensive directory of CSAs, there are currently more than 2,500 CSAs listed. The way these programs work is quite simple:

- Farmers grow and offer a certain number of "shares" to the public. A share is simply a specified amount of produce based on what's available and is the same for every CSA member. Members generally don't get to choose which produce they receive, so you should be flexible and willing to eating a variety of produce.
- Generally, a share includes a box of fruits and vegetables. However, depending on the type of farm participating in the CSA, other products like eggs, homemade bread, flowers, meat, cheese, and dairy may be offered.
- Interested consumers contact the farm to purchase a membership or subscription for the upcoming season's produce.
- Once the growing season begins and produce is harvested, participating members will receive a share of seasonal produce (in a bag, box, or basket) each week throughout the growing season.
- Members may either pick up their shares directly from the farm or from a specified CSA drop-off point each week.

WHAT IS A FARMER'S MARKET?

A farmer's market is a special place where the community, the local farmer, and fresh, natural produce come together. Farmer's markets, also commonly referred to as open-air markets, green markets, or street markets, are the hub for "farm to table" connections. These direct-to-consumer relationships allow farmers to sell their products directly to consumers while offering customers an easy and cost-effective way to get their hands on some of freshest, most nutritious natural food in town.

Another added bonus is that farmer's market food is good for the earth. According to the Center for Urban Education about Sustainable Agriculture (CUESA), the average American meal travels about 1,500 miles from farm to table. The shipping involved in getting that food to our kitchens creates carbon emissions that contribute to global warming.

Once you've experienced the ambience of a farmer's market, your approach to eating local is sure to change. I love the sights and smells of fresh produce and just-picked flowers. I smile at the sounds of vibrant conversations and heartfelt laughter. The attraction of farmer's markets brings together people in the community, ignites new relationships, rekindles old acquaintances, and connects us with our food. One of the most worthy activities that goes on at a farmer's market is public education, especially of our youth, about where our food comes from. After all, tomatoes don't come from a can—they come from the land.

But beware: Not all farmer's markets are true to the spirit of eating local. That's why it's important to be a savvy shopper, not only at the grocery store but at the farmer's market as well. Learn what produce is in season for your local area by checking with your state agriculture department for a listing of produce by season. If you happen to see produce at your local market that isn't in season, say blueberries in North Carolina in late fall, you have cause for suspicion. It's likely the vendor purchased the blueberries and perhaps other produce from wholesalers in another region. This means the product you're buying isn't at its peak freshness because of the travel time involved with transit. If you're concerned about a particular item, ask the farmer where the produce was grown and how it reached your town. If the food was shipped in from another location, buying from that vendor will defeat your intention to eat local.

FOUR SMART SHOPPING TIPS

The following four tips will arm you with the information you need to be a smart farmer's market shopper.

1. *Go early and often.* For me, there's nothing more enjoyable than sneaking out of our house on an early Saturday morning, while my husband and son are still sleeping, to meander through our downtown farmer's markets. I love the crisp air, the stillness of the morning, and the uninterrupted personal time my weekly excursions offer me. But apart from that, early shoppers get the freshest produce and the best selection. Plus, the farmers can spend more time answering your questions without the snarls of waiting customers in line behind you!

2. *Take time to browse.* Farmer's markets are brimming with amazing sights, sounds, tastes, and smells waiting for you to explore. This is one trip where you don't want to be pressed for time. I usually take a casual stroll throughout the entire market, stopping briefly at each stand to see what they have to offer that day. Some vendors have become acquaintances, so I always stop by for a brief chat or just wave if they're busy with customers. A few vendors offer tasting samples, which is a good way for you try before you buy. Think about what produce you need at home as well as and which new varieties you would like to try. Always make a point to go home with a new fruit or vegetable each week, as it's a great way to increase the variety of good foods in your diet.

3. *Carry cash.* Many farmer's markets are small-scale business operations without credit card machines. Additionally, not all stands have access to electricity. Don't limit your opportunity to go home with field-fresh produce because the only cash you have is the change you scrape up from the bottom of your purse or pocket. Stop by the ATM machine before you head to the market for the cash you'll need for a morning of shopping. You won't need much money. Farmer's markets offer an affordable way for families to buy organic and local produce.

4. *Take your cooler.* Peak season for farmer's markets is during the warm summer months. You're buying the freshest and most nutritious produce you can buy for your family, so treat it with the utmost care. Carry a cooler in your car, lightly packed with ice, to keep your produce safe and at its peak. A good rule

of thumb is to keep a collapsible cooler in your trunk, so no matter when you feel the urge to swing by the market, you'll be prepared. You can purchase some ice from a local convenience store for the ride home.

Shopping at farmer's markets and participating in CSAs ensures your family will have access to the best produce available, while also saving money and supporting the local farm economy. Learn where your food comes from, shop wisely for the best in food, and relish in the joy of eating local, natural and healthy.

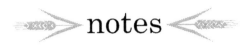# notes